dermatologic radiotherapy

O. BRAUN-FALCO   H. GOLDSCHMIDT

S. LUKACS

dermatologic radiotherapy

WITH 48 ILLUSTRATIONS INCLUDING 16 COLOR PLATES

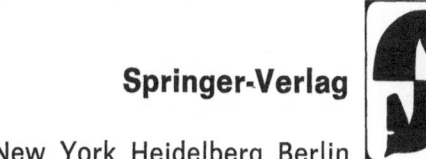
Springer-Verlag

New York Heidelberg Berlin

Otto Braun-Falco, M.D.
Direktor der Dermatologischen
Klinik u. Poliklinik der Universität München
München

Herbert Goldschmidt, M.D.
Suite 620
One Decker Square
Bala-Cynwyd, Pennsylvania 19004

Stefan Lukacs, M.D.
Oberarzt an der Dermatologischen Klinik und
  Poliklinik der Universität München
München

Library of Congress Cataloging in Publication Data

Braun-Falco, Otto, 1922–
    Dermatologic radiotherapy.

    Translation and Revision of Dermatologische Röntgentherapie.
    Bibliography: p. 140
    Includes index.
    1. Skin–Diseases–Radiotherapy. I. Lukacs, Stefan,
joint author. II. Goldschmidt, Herbert, joint author.
III. Title.
RL113.B7313   616.5'064'22   76–44907

© 1976 by Springer-Verlag New York Inc.
Softcover reprint of the hardcover 1st edition 1976

ISBN-13: 978-1-4612-9882-3   e-ISBN-13: 978-1-4612-9880-9
DOI: 10.1007/978-1-4612-9880-9

preface

Ionizing radiation has played an important role in the treatment of skin diseases for many decades. With strict adherence to modern standards of radiation protection, radiotherapy is a safe and effective method that benefits many patients who cannot be treated adequately by other means. Although indications for dermatologic radiotherapy have decreased significantly due to advances in other therapeutic modalities, many dermatologists feel strongly that ionizing radiation is an integral part of dermatologic therapy that should not be relinquished to other specialties because of the highly specialized anatomic, pathologic, and technologic knowledge required. A recent survey of the National Program for Dermatology showed that 44% of 2,444 responding dermatologists use radiotherapy regularly for various skin conditions, particularly in the treatment of cutaneous carcinomas. Significantly, the American Board of Dermatology has decided to continue its requirement of special knowledge in dermatologic radiation therapy for board certification.

Because I have taught this dermatologic subspecialty at various levels, both in Europe and in the United States, I readily agreed to accept Professor Braun-Falco's invitation to cooperate with him and Dr. Lukacs in the preparation of the English edition of this new guide. The text deals mostly with modern concepts of dermatologic radiotherapy and emphasizes practical aspects of treatment. Although it is written as an introduction for young dermatologists, it may also be useful to experienced clinicians who want to keep up with recent developments in this field.

A brief discussion of physical and technological data is included to help the reader understand the proper selection of physical factors. Fundamental radiobiologic concepts and radiation sequelae are also considered. Special emphasis is given to indications for radiotherapy and to its advantages and disadvantages in comparison to other treatment modalities.

Wherever possible the original text has been followed in this English edition. Some sections were abbreviated or eliminated, others were reorganized or extended and some chapters were added to adapt the contents to the needs of the American or British reader. A special effort was made to include pertinent references both from the American and the European literature.

I am grateful to Professor R. Gorson for his review of the chapter on radiation physics and to my secretary, Mrs. M. Sommar, for typing the manuscript. I owe special thanks to my wife, Wiltrud, for the translation of the original text; without her active help, patience, and understanding this work would not have been possible.

Philadelphia, March 1975   Herbert Goldschmidt

acknowledgments

FOR THE GERMAN EDITION

The authors wish to thank Dr. G. Drexler and Dr. W. Panzer (Neuherberg) for their help in the preparation of the physical data, and Dr. K. R. Trott (Munich) for assistance in the chapter on radiobiology. We are particularly grateful to Professor F. Wachsmann for permission to use some of his illustrations. Our photographer, Mr. Bilek, prepared the photographs and drawings.

Otto Braun-Falco

Munich, May 1973

Stefan Lukacs

contents

chapter 2
general radiobiology   45

chapter 5
radiotherapy of benign dermatoses   113

Contents

chapter 6
teleroentgen therapy of generalized
dermatoses   135

bibliography   140

index   146

1

Physical basis of
dermatologic radiotherapy

1.1 ELECTROMAGNETIC RADIATION

X-rays are part of the electromagnetic spectrum, which also includes gamma rays, ultraviolet light, visible light, infrared light, and radio waves. Electromagnetic waves are a form of energy; other forms are kinetic, thermal, nuclear, and gravitational energy. They may be described as the periodic variation of intensities of electric and magnetic fields at a given point (Selman 1960; Johns and Cunningham 1969). Electromagnetic waves travel in a straight line from their source and are independent of the presence of matter. They are characterized by the following parameters:

1. The frequency (ν) is the number of waves passing a given point each second, or the number of vibrations per second.
2. The wavelength (λ) is the distance between two successive points in the wave that are characterized by the same phase of oscillation.
3. The velocity (c) is the distance the wave moves per second; it is a function of the frequency of the radiation and of the nature of the medium traversed. (In a vacuum or in air, all electromagnetic waves move at a speed of 299,793 km/sec, or 186,171 miles/sec.)

The relationship among frequency, wavelength, and velocity is expressed by the equation:

$$c = \nu\lambda$$

1

In order to understand such processes as emission and absorption, and such concepts as energy and intensity of radiation, we must think of electromagnetic radiation (especially roentgen and gamma radiation) as consisting of both waves and discrete energy particles, known as photons or quanta. The energy of a quantum is given by the equation:

$$E = h\nu$$

where E is the energy in ergs, h is a universal constant (Planck's constant or "element of action," having the magnitude 6.625×10^{-27} erg–sec), and ν is the frequency of the electromagnetic wave.

The unit of energy most often used in radiologic physics is the electron volt (eV), which is defined as the kinetic energy acquired by an electron falling unimpeded through a potential difference of 1 V and is equivalent to 1.602×10^{-12} erg or 1.6×10^{-19} J (Table 1).

TABLE 1

WAVELENGTHS AND PHOTON ENERGIES OF ELECTROMAGNETIC RADIATIONS

Type of radiation	Wavelength	Photon energy
Radio	3×10^5 to 1 cm	4×10^{-10} to 1.2×10^{-4} eV
Infrared	50 to 0.75 μ	0.025 to 1.6 eV
Visible light	760 to 400 mμ	1.6 to 3.0 eV
Ultraviolet	400 to 100 mμ	3.0 to 12 eV
X rays	1 to 0.01 Å (and less)	10 to 1000 keV (and up)

1.2 PRODUCTION OF X RAYS

X rays are produced when high-speed electrons strike matter; this may occur in one of two ways:

Bremsstrahlung

An electron having the energy E_{kin} enters the electric field of an atomic nucleus and is deflected from its original path. This induces the electron to yield up a fraction of its energy in the form of an x-ray quantum having the energy $h\nu$. The resultant loss of kinetic energy causes deceleration of the electron, which now has the energy $E_{kin} - h\nu$. The roentgen radiation produced by this braking effect is called *bremsstrahlung* or brems radiation (i.e., braking radiation). (See Fig. 1.) The probability of this process taking place increases and the brems-ray effect becomes more pronounced

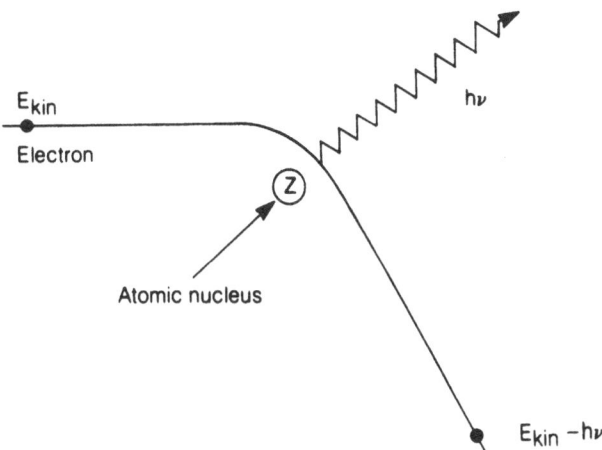

Figure 1. Production of brems radiation.

as the atomic number (Z) of the target element is increased. The greater the deflection of the electron from its original course, the higher will be the energy $h\nu$ of the brems-ray quantum emitted. In the limiting case, the entire kinetic energy of the electron is converted to a brems-ray quantum, $h\nu = E_{kin}$. The spectrum of the brems radiation thus produced is continuous, including the entire energy range from $h\nu = 0$ to $h\nu = E_{kin}$; hence, the initial energy of the incident electron represents the upper limit of the energy of the brems-ray spectrum emitted. The initial kinetic energy of the electron is a function of the magnitude of the applied voltage. For example, in an x-ray tube having a voltage of 40 kV (or 40,000 V), the electrons acquire an energy of 40 keV (or 40,000 eV), according to the definition of the electron volt given above (Figs. 1 and 2).

Characteristic Radiation

Upon collision with a high-speed electron, an orbital electron may be dislodged from its inner orbit and jump to an outer shell not filled to capacity; this transition from a lower to a higher level of energy puts the atom in a state of excitation. Likewise, the orbital electron may be ejected completely from the atom—a process resulting in ionization (see Fig. 2).

Both states are unstable; a return to the stable ground state is achieved by an orbital electron from an outer shell moving into the space vacated by the inner orbital electron. This displacement is associated with emission of one or more photons. The energy $h\nu$ of such a photon or quantum is characteristic of the atom and hence of the element in which the process is taking place; the radiation produced in this manner is therefore called

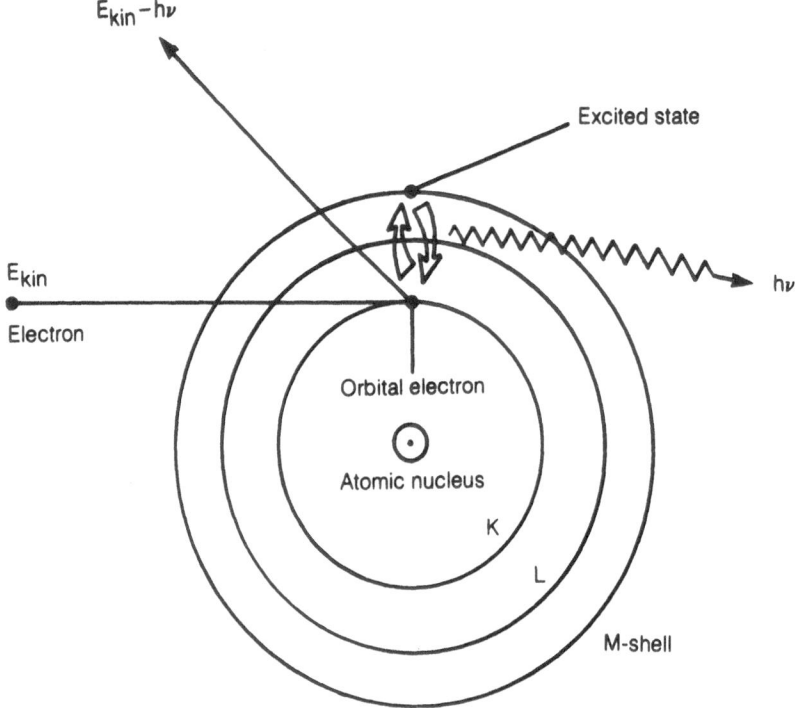

Figure 2. Production of characteristic radiation.

characteristic radiation. Thus, replacement of an electron on the K orbit results in emission of the characteristic K radiation of an element, while replacement of an electron on the L orbit produces characteristic L radiation, etc.

The process of x-ray production by displacement of an orbital electron requires the following conditions:

1. The target element must have a high atomic number (e.g., tungsten); only then are the energies of the photons produced by replacement of inner orbital electrons high enough to fall into the range of x radiation. Use of elements with a lower atomic number would result in less energetic (e.g., ultraviolet) radiation.

2. The energy of the incident high-speed electron must be greater than the binding energy holding the orbital electrons in their inner shells (e.g., K and L). In order to dislodge an electron on the K orbit of tungsten, an energy of >67 keV is required; this means that the x-ray tube must have a

voltage of at least 67 kV. A voltage of about 12 kV is sufficient to excite *L* radiation.

The efficiency of x-ray production by either of the two processes described above is very low, however. The majority of the high-speed electrons lose their kinetic energy in collisions with outer orbital electrons, a process that merely imparts heat to the target material. At 100 kV, less than 1% of the energy applied to accelerate the high-speed electrons is converted to x radiation, whereas more than 99% is converted to heat.

1.3   THE X-RAY TUBE

A schematic representation of an x-ray tube is given in Fig. 3. A spiral of tungsten wire is heated by a filament heating current of several amperes; by the process of thermionic emission, electrons are liberated from the filament that constitutes the cathode of the x-ray tube. The stream of electrons is then condensed into a narrow beam by means of a focusing device and accelerated by the high voltage applied between cathode (filament) and anode (target). The flow of high-speed electrons driven toward the anode constitutes the tube current (several milliamperes). The tube voltages used in dermatologic radiation therapy generally are below 50 kV but may reach 100 kV. The cathode stream of high-speed electrons

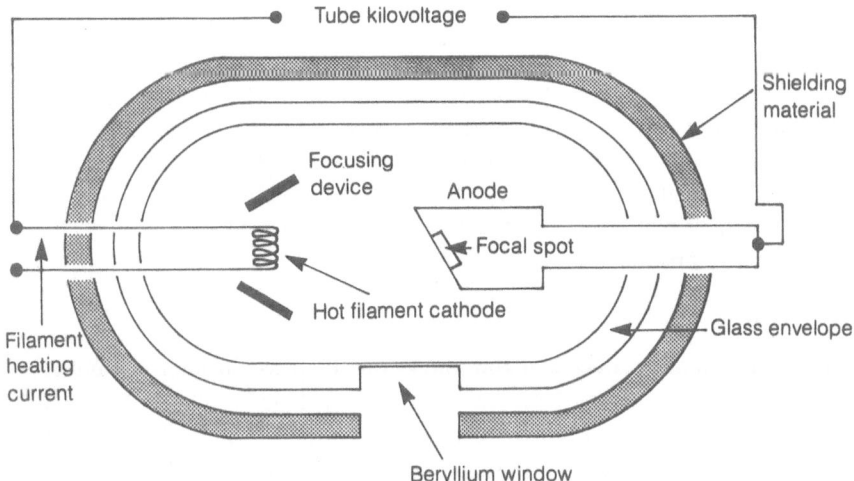

Figure 3.   Schematic diagram of x-ray tube.

strikes the target, i.e., the focal spot of the anode, which in therapy x-ray tubes has a diameter of about 6 mm. This is where the processes described in paragraph 2 (p. 2) take place. Because the production of x rays is associated with considerable heat production, the focal spot must consist of extremely heat-resistant material—usually tungsten. This tungsten disk is embedded in a good heat conductor, such as copper, which directs the heat away from the anode and toward the cooling system (not shown in Fig. 3). The electrodes are enclosed in a glass chamber containing a high vacuum, which minimizes loss of energy by collision of fast electrons with gas molecules and prevents oxidation of the filament by residual gas.

Because the penetrating power of the radiation used in dermatologic radiation therapy is low, the exit portal of the tube must consist of a material that attenuates x rays only slightly; in most cases, thin beryllium windows are used. Radiation hitting the inner wall of the tube in places other than the exit portal is absorbed by the glass tube or by the tube cover (Fig. 3).

1.4   RADIATION QUALITY

Factors Affecting Radiation Quality

The quality of an x-ray beam is specified by its spectral distribution curve. The x-ray spectrum includes the brems-ray spectrum and the characteristic x-ray spectrum and is dependent upon the following factors:

TUBE KILOVOLTAGE

As indicated on page 3, the kilovoltage applied to the tube determines the upper limit of the energy range of the brems-ray spectrum. The applied kilovoltage also determines whether and to what extent characteristic radiation is excited in the x-ray tube. A third function of the kilovoltage is the depth of penetration of the fast electrons, and hence the exact location of x-ray production within the target.

FILTRATION

The x-ray beam produced in the anode has to pass through a number of layers before it emerges from the x-ray tube. This results in attenuation of the original beam and also—because the attenuation is energy dependent—in a change in the original spectral distribution. Such layers are:

- The layer between the site of production of the x-ray beam and the surface of the focal spot: This inherent absorption of the anode is responsible for the so-called "heel effect," which results in nonuniform irradiation of the field (Fig. 4).

- The exit portal: The attenuation and change in spectral distribution caused by these two layers are called the inherent filtration of the tube.
- Added filtration modifying the radiation quality to suit the purpose of radiation therapy.
- The air between exit portal and a given point within the irradiated field: This is especially important when x rays of low penetrating ability are used.

Figure 5 shows spectra emitted by a beryllium-window tube after application of various kilovoltages and filters. At 100 kV, the characteristic *K* radiation of tungsten is excited, causing sharp peaks at 58 and 68 keV; these *K* lines are superimposed on the continuous brems-ray spectrum, as is the *L* radiation at 10 keV. The latter, however, fails to penetrate the 1.7-mm Al filter, which also absorbs the low-energy portion of the brems-ray spectrum. At 55 kV there is no *K* radiation, and the *L* radiation is absorbed almost completely by 0.8-mm Al. The narrow spectrum produced by a tube kilovoltage of 20 kV is composed of the characteristic *L* radiation and the brems-ray spectrum. There is no clear distinction between the two components.

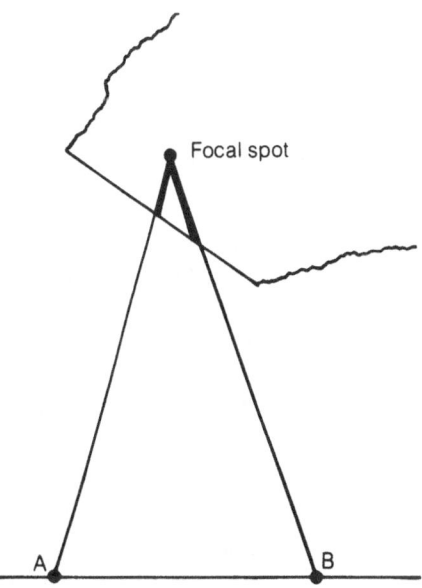

Figure 4. Heel effect: Roentgen radiation originating at the same point within the focal spot has to traverse a greater part of the anode in order to reach point B than in order to reach point A.

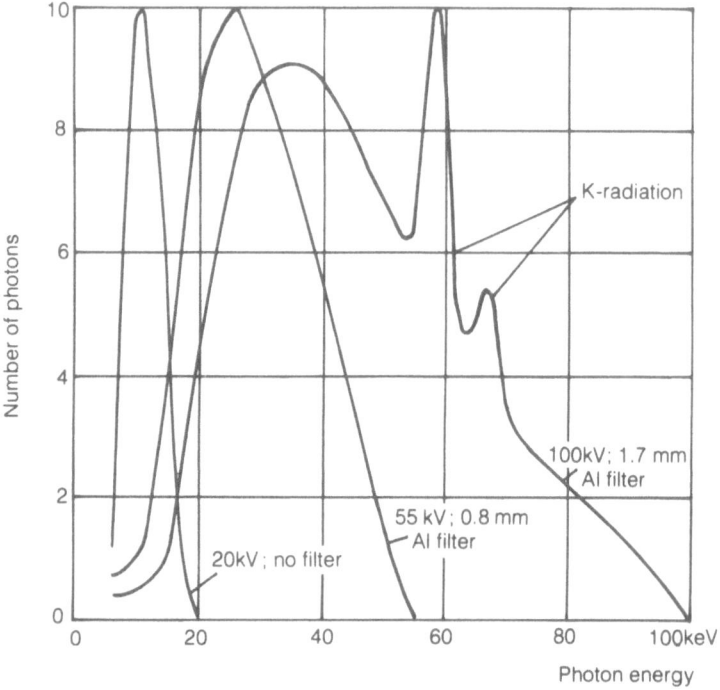

Figure 5. Spectra emitted by a beryllium window tube after application of various kilovoltages and filters.

DEFINITION

The quality of radiation is described completely by its spectral curve. However, spectral determinations require elaborate physical equipment and rather complicated procedures. It is therefore customary in dermatologic radiotherapy to define radiation quality by less precise but—for all practical purposes—entirely adequate parameters. Among these are:

1. Specification of applied kilovoltage and added filtration
2. Specification of penetrating power, or "hardness," of radiation:
   Ultrasoft radiation—tube voltage up to 20 kV
   Soft radiation—tube voltage 20–60 kV
   Superficial radiation—tube voltage 60–150 kV
   (Other radiation qualities are not used in dermatologic practice. "Grenz rays" are produced at 10–20 kV and are therefore classified as ultrasoft radiation.)
3. Specification of half-value layer (HVL) or half-value thickness (HVT) (see p. 10).

1.5   RADIATION QUANTITY

Radiation quantity varies with the magnitude of the tube current (milliamperage) if the applied kilovoltage remains constant. An increase in applied kilovoltage, with the milliamperage remaining constant, not only produces a change in spectral distribution of the quanta emitted but also increases the number of quanta produced.

1.6   INTERACTION OF X RADIATION AND MATTER

Roentgen radiation striking an object produces a change in that object. The nature and duration of that change depend on a variety of factors: the nature of the matter entered by the radiation, the amount and energy of the radiation received, previous treatment of the object, and spacing of dosage, among others. There is an almost unlimited number of possible changes, ranging from relatively simple and predictable processes, such as those used in detecting and measuring radiation, to the complex changes produced in biologic objects. If we limit our discussion to the physical processes involved, the following possibilities may be encountered within the energy range relevant to dermatologic radiation therapy:

1. Transmission (passage through matter unchanged). A photon passes through an object without encounter, emerging unchanged in energy or direction.

2. Absorption. Photoelectric collision with true absorption occurs when a photon gives up all its energy (hv) to an inner orbital electron, which then becomes a photoelectron having the kinetic energy $E_{kin} = hv - E_B$ (E_B is the binding energy of the dislodged orbital electron). This photoelectron moves on through matter, knocking out several thousand orbital electrons and creating excited or ionized atoms along the way, until all its energy is spent. Excitation and ionization by secondary electrons are the primary changes produced by x radiation in matter. The range of penetration of these photoelectrons in tissue is several microns (see Fig. 6).

3. Unmodified scattering. A photon entering an atom is not absorbed but undergoes a change in direction without loss of energy; the matter traversed remains unaltered. This process results in attenuation of the roentgen radiation, because the photons thus affected stray from the original beam and fail to hit the target (Figs. 6 and 7).

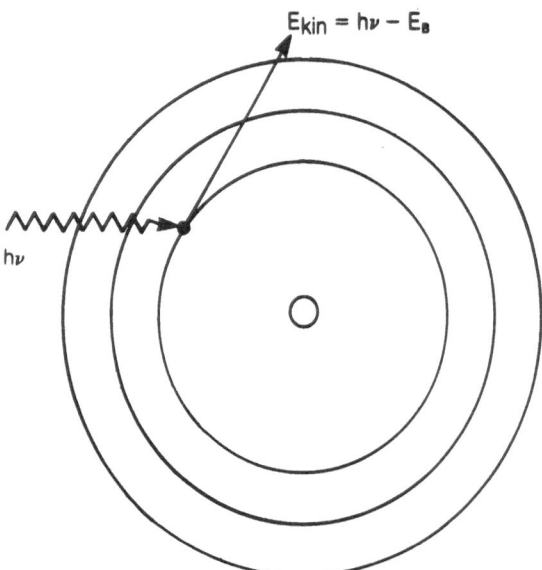

Figure 6. Photoelectric effect.

4. Compton effect. A photon entering matter gives up part of its energy to an outer orbital electron and proceeds with the remainder of its energy in a new direction (modified scattering). The dislodged electron ("Compton" or "recoil" electron) acts in the same manner as a photoelectron, creating ionized atoms along its path until its energy is spent (absorption by scattering). The Compton effect is named for its discoverer, A. H. Compton.

The relative frequency of the processes described above is dependent on the energy of the radiation and nature of the irradiated material. In the case of soft tissue, and within the energy range relevant to radiotherapy, the photoelectric effect (Fig. 6) is predominant up to 30 keV, whereas the Compton effect (Fig. 7) occurs more frequently in the range above 30 keV. With absorbing materials having a high atomic number, the photoelectric effect generally predominates.

Half-Value Layer (HVL); Half-Value Thickness (HVT)

The quality of an x-ray beam at a given point of the irradiated field is specified completely by the relative spectral distribution of the constituent photons. However, because determination of spectral curves is too complicated a procedure to be practical in routine radiotherapy, it has become

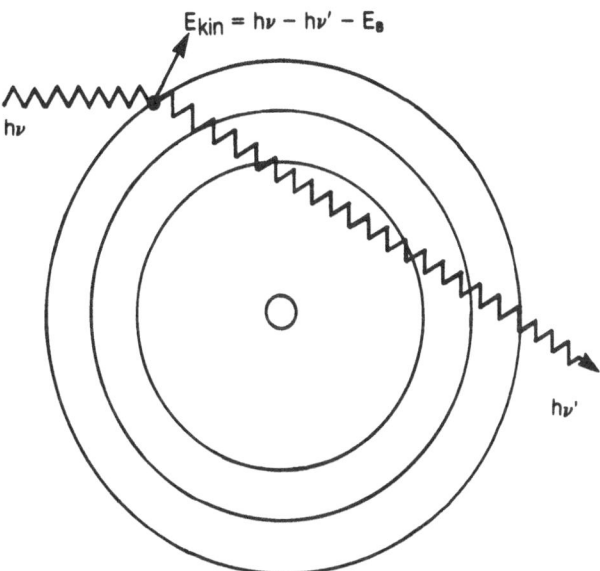

Figure 7. Compton effect.

customary to specify radiation quality in terms of interaction of radiation with certain materials. The first half-value layer (HVL) is that thickness of a given filter material which reduces the intensity of a narrow x-ray beam to 50% of its initial value. The new term "half-value thickness" (HVT) has been proposed to replace the term half-value layer (HVL). At this date, it has not been universally accepted and most publications have continued to use the designation HVL to avoid misinterpretations. The second HVL is the thickness of the same material required to attenuate the x-ray beam another 50% (i.e., from 50% to 25%). The degree of

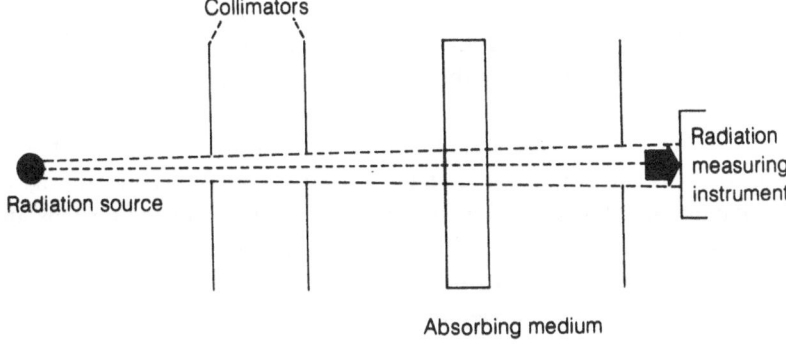

Figure 8. Experimental arrangement to measure absorption of x rays.

11

energy homogeneity is expressed by the ratio of the first to the second HVL (homogeneity factor). A homogeneity factor smaller than 1.0 denotes a heterogeneous radiation, whereas a factor approaching 1.0 denotes a homogeneous radiation.

In dermatologic radiotherapy, aluminum and occasionally tissue-equivalent materials are used as standard HVL materials.

Attenuation

The attenuation of x rays may be determined quantitatively in the following manner: let us consider a collimated beam of specified energy as shown in Fig. 8. N_o represents the original number of photons in the incident beam as recorded by the measuring device without an absorber present; N is the number of photons measured after the beam has passed through an absorber of the thickness x. The relationship between these two quantities may be expressed as follows:

$$N = N_o e - \mu x$$

where μ is the attenuation coefficient, which varies with the energy of the radiation and the atomic number and density of the absorbing material; e is a constant (2.718). The transmission of monoenergetic photons decreases exponentially with increasing thickness of the absorbing material. By inserting an absorber of a thickness that reduces the intensity of the incident beam (N_o) by 50%, we arrive at the definition of the half-value layer (HVL).

An additional half-value layer would reduce N_o to $N_o/4$ (provided the radiation measured is monoenergetic); an absorber consisting of three half-value layers would attenuate the beam to $N_o/8$, etc.

By specifying the HVL of an absorber (e.g., aluminum), we implicitly define the radiation quality used: harder, more penetrating radiation qualities require a greater HVL than do softer qualities. Hence, various radiation qualities may be specified by indicating the appropriate HVL (see p. 11). For this purpose, the measuring instrument must be a standard dosimeter.

When the attenuation of a wide beam by an absorber of extensive thickness is measured, the equation given above is useful only as an approximation. Half-value layers measured under such conditions may be misleading, because radiation that in the absence of an absorber would bypass the measuring instrument may be directed toward the instrument through scattering processes occurring within the absorber.

1.7 RADIATION DOSIMETRY

Basic Concepts

It is the objective of dosimetry to determine the amount of energy deposited by radiation in an absorbing medium, such as biologic tissue. This quantity cannot be measured directly. It may be calculated from the number and energies of incident photons per time and area, for the probabilities for the photoelectric and Compton processes can be determined with relative accuracy; but this is a complicated and time-consuming procedure, and more practical ways have therefore been sought.

EXPOSURE

(Exposure Dose, X) The concept of exposure (X) is based on the ability of electromagnetic radiation to ionize air. The exposure specifies the amount of ionization produced in a small mass of air around a point of interest under certain defined conditions of measurement. The special unit of the radiation exposure is the roentgen (R), which may be defined as that quantity of x rays or gamma rays which produces 1 esu (electrostatic unit) of electricity of either sign in 1 cm³ of air, or 2.58×10^{-4} coulombs (C) per kg, or 86.9 ergs/g (air).

A device capable of measuring radiation quantity in terms of ionization in air is the free air ionization chamber. In this instrument, a quantity of x rays is passed through a segregated volume of air. The liberated ions are collected and the quantity of electricity carried by them is measured. The chamber must be designed so as to allow as many secondary electrons to enter the segregated volume of air as leave it, in order to have electronic equilibrium.

The *exposure rate* is the intensity of radiation at a given point in the beam; it is stated in roentgens per unit time (exposure/time), usually roentgen/minutes.

ABSORBED DOSE (D)

The absorbed dose (D) is the amount of energy absorbed per unit mass of specified material (tissue, bone, etc.) at a point of interest from any directly or indirectly ionizing radiation. The special unit of the absorbed dose is the rad; 1 rad represents an absorbed dose of 100 ergs/g tissue, or 10^{-2} J/kg. The *absorbed dose rate* is stated in rads per unit time, usually rads/minutes. The ratio of absorbed dose to exposure (rads/roentgen) may be expressed by means of a quantity often referred to as the roentgen to rads conversion factor (f):

$$f(Z,E) = D/X \ (\text{rads/R})$$

The number of rads of absorbed dose per roentgen of exposure depends on the atomic number (Z) of the irradiated material and the energy (E) of the x rays.

In Fig. 9 the f factor has been calculated for various tissues and photon energies of interest to radiotherapists.

DOSE EQUIVALENT (H)

The biologic effect of radiation is not only a function of the energy absorbed, but also of the type of radiation used. Equal doses of energy, produced by x rays in one instance and by neutrons in another, differ considerably in biologic effectiveness. To account for this difference in response, especially for purposes of radiation protection, a quality factor (q) has been introduced, which is based on the concept of relative biologic

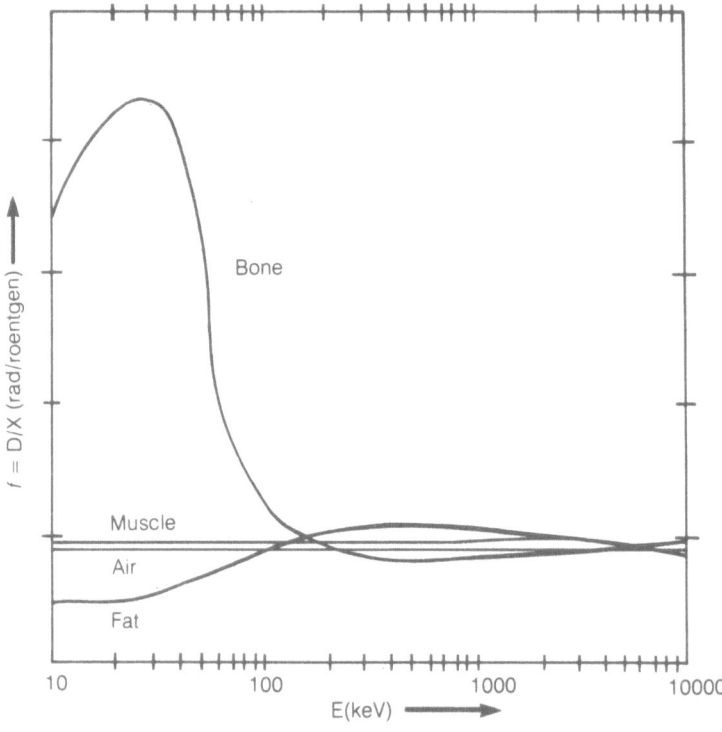

Figure 9. Ratio of absorbed dose (**D**) to exposure (**X**) as a function of energy for various tissues.

effectiveness (RBE). The latter may be defined as the inverse ratio of the absorbed dose from one radiation type to that of a reference radiation required to produce the same degree of a stipulated effect. With x rays, gamma rays, and beta rays as reference radiation, the following values for q are obtained:

Radiation type	q
Roentgen, gamma, beta	1
Alpha, protons	10
Neutrons	3–10
Deuterons, recoil nuclei	20

Use of the term "dose equivalent" (H) is limited to statements concerning radiation protection. The unit of H is the rem. H may be expressed numerically as the absorbed dose in rads multiplied by the quality factor: H (rem) $= D$ (rad) q. (Whereas RBE is always experimentally determined, the quality factor q is assigned on the basis of a number of considerations.)

INVERSE SQUARE LAW

According to the inverse square law, which applies to all forms of radiation emitted uniformly from a point source, the intensity of radiation at a given distance from the source is inversely proportional to the square of the distance. If the radiation intensity at distance a from the focal spot is I_1, the radiation intensity I_2 at distance b may be calculated from the following equation (provided there are no absorbing or scattering media between these two points):

$$I_2 = I_1 \cdot \frac{a^2}{b^2}$$

Thus, if the distance is doubled ($b = 2a$), the resulting intensity I_2 becomes $1/4$ of the initial intensity I_1; tripling of the distance results in a decrease of the intensity to $1/9$ of I_1, etc. Inverse square proportion may also be expressed geometrically as shown in Fig. 10.

Special Concepts

In addition to the quantities defined in the preceding paragraph, a number of special quantities and units have been introduced and found useful in radiotherapeutic practice. Because some of these quantities are linked to certain defined conditions of measurement, a brief description seems in order. The preferred units of radiation dosage are the rad (sometimes rd),

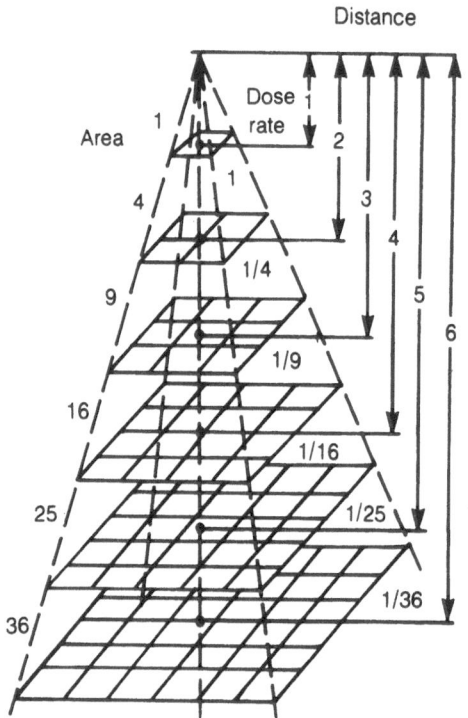

Figure 10. Diagram showing decrease of radiation intensity with the distance squared (modified from Wachsmann and Vieten 1970).

which is the special unit of the absorbed dose, and the roentgen, which is the special unit of exposure.

- *Incident* or *air dose*. The exposure in roentgens produced under specified conditions (tube kilovoltage, milliamperage, added filtration, collimator, field size), as measured in air on the central axis of the beam at a given target–skin distance (TSD) by means of an ionization chamber.
- *Backscatter*. The radiation dose scattered back from the irradiated medium to the surface, thus adding to the incident dose. Backscatter may be expressed in percent of the incident dose or as the ratio of the skin dose (see below) to incident dose (backscatter factor).
- *Surface dose* (skin dose). The radiation dose absorbed in tissue at a point of the surface of the body; hence, the skin dose is the sum of the incident dose and the backscatter dose at the surface.
- *Depth dose*. The radiation dose at a specified depth of the irradiated body as measured under specified conditions.

- *Relative depth dose (percentage depth dose).* The depth dose relative to the skin dose.
- *Tissue dose.* The absorbed dose at a specified point of the treatment volume.
- *Integral dose.* The mean energy imparted ($\bar{\epsilon}$) or the expectation value of the energy imparted by ionizing radiation to the matter in a volume.
- *Specific energy imparted* (z). The quotient of ϵ by m, where ϵ is the energy imparted by ionizing radiation to the matter in a volume element and m is the mass of the matter in that volume element. The special unit of specific energy imparted is the rad.

Basic Methods

The most widely used method of dosage determination in radiotherapy is that of measuring the ionization produced in a specific amount of air or gas. The dosimeters used for the calibration of x-ray machines consist of the following main components:

1. An ionization chamber (free air or walled) containing two electrodes. (In walled chambers, the wall serves as one electrode and the other is placed centrally.)
2. A voltage source for the application of a potential difference between the two electrodes.
3. An electric measuring device (electrometer) for indicating the amount of ionization produced in the chamber.

Radiation exposure may be expressed as air dose (incident dose), skin dose (surface dose), or absorbed dose (tissue dose). For calibration purposes, determination of the air dose is the most convenient method. The primary standard for the measurement of x-ray exposure in roentgens is the standard free air ionization chamber, against which other (smaller and simpler) instruments must be calibrated. A practical instrument for use in clinical work is the condenser R meter (Victoreen meter), which consists of a thimble chamber and a charging and measuring system. In the thimble chamber, the "air wall" of the standard ionization chamber has been replaced by a wall of solid material (e.g., plastic) that is air equivalent, i.e., that has the same effective atomic number as air (7.7). For the measurement of soft x rays, conventional thimble chambers are inadequate because of wall absorption. Therefore, special thin-walled ionization chambers have been developed which are made of nylon (about 0.05 mm in thickness). These instruments are highly useful for calibrating x-ray machines equipped with beryllium-window tubes.

17

SENSITIVITY AND ACCURACY OF THE IONIZATION CHAMBER

Accurate readings of the dose or dose rate within a given range of radiation quality can be obtained only if the ionization chamber is calibrated specifically for that range or if it is energy independent over a fairly wide range. The relative sensitivity of two types of ionization chambers as a function of radiation quality is shown in Fig. 11. As the figure illustrates, a thimble chamber can be used in soft radiation therapy only if the radiation quality is known precisely, whereas a thin-walled chamber records measurements within the range of interest that are independent of radiation quality (Fig. 11). Appropriate corrections must be made for angle of incidence, temperature, atmospheric pressure, and chamber energy dependence. Correction factors can be obtained from tables furnished with the instrument. The maximum dose rate stated by the manufacturer must not be exceeded. The chamber and electrometer must be recalibrated periodically.

Dosimeters Commonly Used in Dermatologic Radiation Therapy

- Victoreen dosimeter, model 651. Low-energy chamber with a thin Mylar end window.

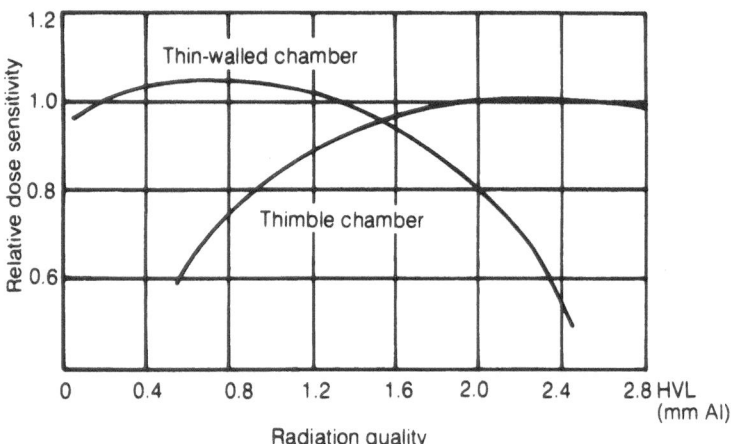

Figure 11. Schematic representation of the relative sensitivity of two types of ionization chambers as a function of energy (courtesy of Dr. G. Drexler, Institute of Radiation Protection, Neuherberg, Germany).

- Siemens dosimeter. Special chambers for soft x-ray therapy are available.
- Farmer dosimeter (Nuclear Enterprises, Lighthill, Edinburgh, Scotland). Battery operated; equipped with a number of interchangeable ionization chambers. For dermatologic purposes, a thin-walled chamber using Perspex (skin-equivalent material) as scattering material is available; energy independent from 10 kV, HVL 0.038 mm Al, to 100 kV, HVL 2 mm Al.
- Universal dosimeter (Philips). May be switched from dose to dose rate; special soft ray and phantom chambers available.
- Simplex dosimeter (Phys.-Tech. Werkstätten, Freiburg; available through Nuclear Associates, Westbury, N.Y.).

Frequency of Calibration

An x-ray therapy unit must be calibrated on installation and periodically thereafter—usually once a year. A complete calibration should be made after repair or replacement of any part of the machine that may affect the dose rate. If possible, the calibrations should be performed by a certified radiologic physicist. The dosimeter used for calibration must be checked periodically for accuracy and constancy of both chamber and electrometer.

Procedure of Dose Measurement

In soft radiation therapy, measurement of air dose and skin dose by means of thin-walled ionization chambers as shown in Figs. 12 and 13 is the most commonly used method.

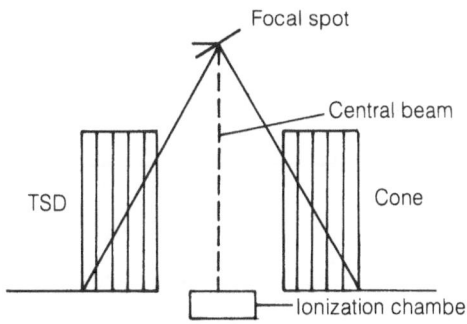

Figure 12. Determination of air dose.

19

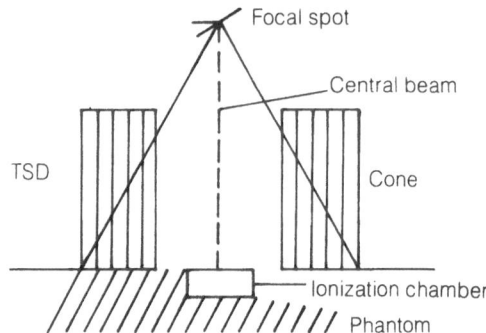

Figure 13. Determination of skin dose.

Determination of the air dose should be made at the TSD employed, in order to account for absorption in air. If cones are used, this method also accounts for scattering. The reading obtained is multiplied by the backscatter factor (Fig. 14). The product of air dose and backscatter factor represents the skin dose. Determination of the skin dose can be made directly, as shown in Fig. 13. Extrapolation chambers and tissue-equivalent

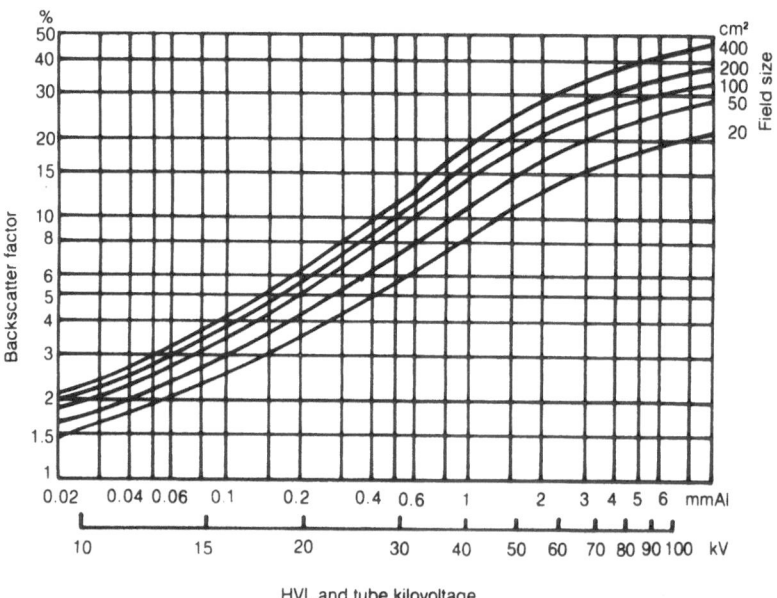

Figure 14. Backscatter as a function of radiation quality and field size (modified from Wachsmann and Dimotsis 1957).

ionization chambers are available that eliminate the need for a separate phantom and record true energy absorption.

Measurement of Dose Distribution in the Body

In radiotherapy, measurement of the incident dose or skin dose is only the first step in treatment planning; subsequent steps are:

1. Determination of dose distribution (relative depth dose) under specified treatment conditions
2. Variation of the treatment conditions in order to achieve optimal dose distribution; i.e., to maximize the amount of absorbed dose in the region occupied by the lesion and to minimize the dose to adjacent normal tissue
3. Selection of exposure time
4. Control measurements

HALF-VALUE DEPTH ($D_{1/2}$).

The half-value depth (HVD or $D_{1/2}$) is the depth in tissue at which the dose is 50% of the surface dose (skin dose) (Wachsmann 1950; Jennings 1951; Tuddenham 1957). In planning the therapy of superficial lesions, one should give as large a dose as necessary to the lesion and as little as possible to the underlying tissue. This may be expressed by a simple relation between $D_{1/2}$ and depth of the lesion: in order to obtain a maximum value for the ratio of energy absorbed within the pathologic layer (L) to total energy absorbed, one should aim for conditions approximating

$$D_{1/2} = 0.7 \times L$$

This rule may be varied to suit individual requirements, from $D_{1/2} = 0.3 \times L$ to $D_{1/2} = 1.5 \times L$.

> *Rule of Thumb:* The $D_{1/2}$ should approximate the depth of the lesion ($D_{1/2} = L$) (Schirren 1959).

The half-value depth as a parameter of radiation quality is influenced by the following variables (Fig. 15a, b):

a. Tube kilovoltage
b. Total filtration (inherent filtration, added filtration; in certain cases, filtration by air)
c. Target–skin distance
d. Field size and shape.

The relationship between tube kilovoltage, filtration, and $D_{1/2}$ at an

21

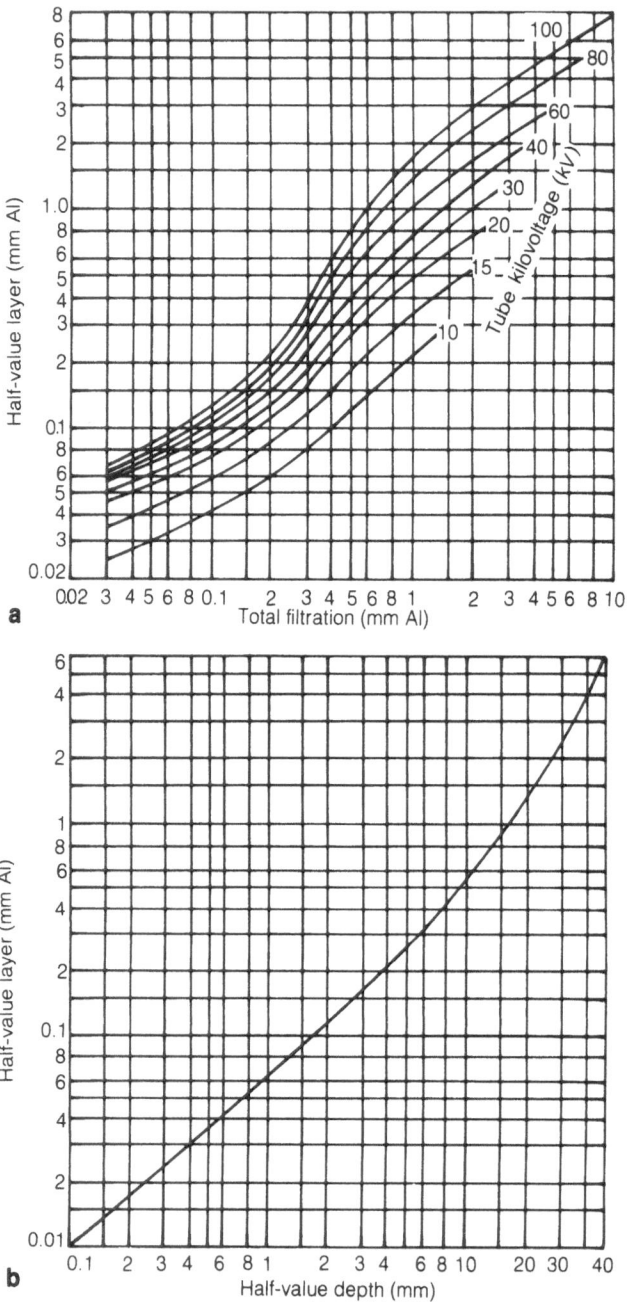

Figure 15. **a.** Half-value layer (HVL) of soft radiation as a function of filtration (modified from Wachsmann 1959). **b.** Relationship between HVL and $D_{1/2}$ at a target–skin distance of 30 cm and a field diameter of ca. 100 cm.

approximately constant dose rate is shown in Fig. 15a and b. By describing the parameters kilovoltage and filtration in terms of half-value layer (HVL) of the radiation (Fig. 15a), a relationship between HVL and $D_{1/2}$ is established (Fig. 15b).

The effect of the TSD on the relative depth dose is primarily of a geometric nature and is based on the inverse square law (see p. 15). The dosage difference obtained at a TSD of 20 cm versus one of 30 cm is:

$$\frac{20^2}{30^2} = 56\%$$

whereas at a TSD of 70 cm versus one of 80 cm the dosage difference is only:

$$\frac{70^2}{80^2} = 23\%$$

It is important to note that the increase in $D_{1/2}$ associated with an increase in TSD is not because of a change in radiation quality but because at a greater TSD the depth dose is greater in relation to the surface dose (see Fig. 16).

Another factor that has to be considered in soft-ray therapy is the absorption of radiation in air. The diagram in Fig. 17 illustrates the effect on the $D_{1/2}$ of the physical factors mentioned above. It also shows how increased scattering at increasing field size changes the $D_{1/2}$ (Fig. 17).

Irradiation of multiple adjacent fields may result in overlapping, which may considerably alter the depth–dose curve. However, with the relatively great target–skin distances used in modern soft x-ray therapy it is possible to irradiate even large areas as a single field.

> *Rule of Thumb:* The TSD should be twice the diameter of the irradiated area.

Because accurate dosimetry and responsible treatment planning require experience as well as familiarity with physical concepts, it is advisable to consult a radiologic physicist in these matters.

1.8   SELECTION OF PHYSICAL TREATMENT FACTORS

In modern dermatologic radiation therapy there is a tendency to standardize treatment techniques and to reduce variations of physical factors to a minimum in order to eliminate technical and human errors. This aim can be achieved with modern x-ray units (Wachsmann 1959; Goldschmidt 1959, 1976).

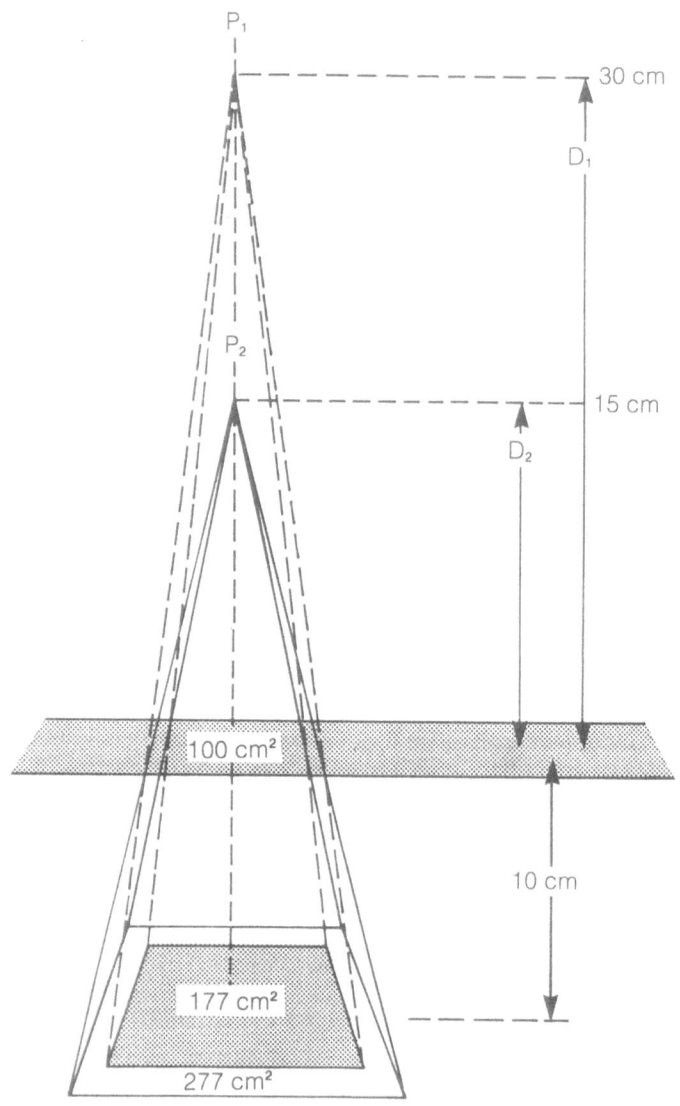

Figure 16. Diagram illustrating the reason for greater depth dose with greater target–skin distance. The area irradiated at 10 cm below the surface from the greater target–skin distance (P_1) is 177 cm², while that irradiated from the shorter target–skin distance (P_2) is 277 cm². The same amount of radiation applied to the surface area of 100 cm² is spread more sparsely over the area which is 277 cm² in size (from Cipollaro and Crossland 1967).

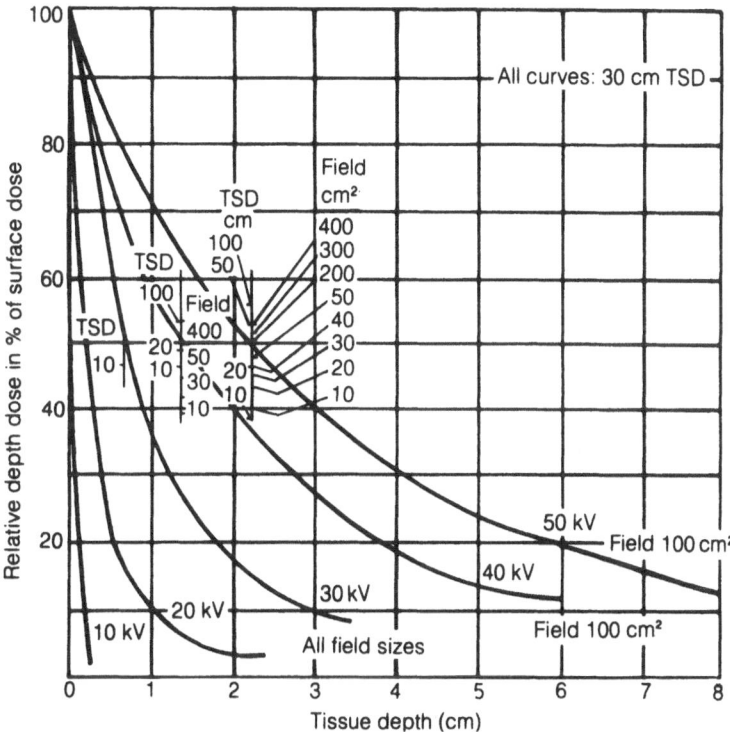

Figure 17. Depth doses of soft radiation at 30 cm TSD and 100 cm² field size. For comparison, the effect of variations in field size and TSD is also shown (modified from Wachsmann and Dimotsis 1957).

Factors Affecting Radiation Quality

TUBE KILOVOLTAGE

The quality, or penetrating ability, of the radiation varies with the tube kilovoltage, which in dermatologic radiation therapy may range from about 10 to about 100 kV.

FILTRATION

Filters are used in x-ray therapy to enhance the homogeneity or penetration of the radiation. Selection of filters should be governed by the following recommendations:

1. In general, only aluminum filters are used.
2. Manufacturers usually supply only three to five standard filters (e.g., 0.25, 0.5, 1.0, or 2.0 mm Al).

25

3. In dermatologic office practice, three to five combinations of kilovoltages and filters are usually sufficient.

When technically feasible, the combinations of kilovoltage and filtration should be arranged to yield the same dose rate for different radiation qualities in order to reduce the margin of error. In some modern units, the selection of kilovoltage and filtration is monitored by interlock devices that virtually eliminate the possibility of error.

TARGET–SKIN DISTANCE (TSD)

It is advisable to standardize the TSD as much as possible and to regulate dosage falloff primarily by varying the radiation quality instead of by varying the TSD. Because the use of cones is advised for most therapeutic purposes, the selection of the proper TSD is limited to the TSD of the cones supplied with the radiation unit. Most manufacturers supply only cones of two lengths: either 15 and 30 cm or 20 and 40 cm TSD. In addition to limiting unnecessary variations of the TSD, the use of cones also insures accurate target–skin distances.

> *Rule of Thumb:* The TSD should be at least twice the diameter of the irradiated area.

Disadvantages of a very short TSD:

1. Only small areas can be irradiated.
2. Curved or uneven surfaces cannot be irradiated uniformly.

Factors Affecting Radiation Quantity

TUBE CURRENT (mA)

With most modern x-ray machines the settings for amperage are limited to those recommended by the manufacturer (e.g., 5 mA, 25 mA). Variations are not required.

TARGET–SKIN DISTANCE (TSD)

Variations in TSD produce changes in dose rate according to the inverse square law (see p. 15). Absorption in air has to be considered when soft radiation qualities are used.

FIELD SIZE

EFFECT ON SKIN DOSE BY WAY OF BACKSCATTER

With the radiation qualities used in dermatologic radiation therapy, backscatter is significant only when more penetrating radiation qualities are used for large field sizes. The backscatter factor may be 0.3 for a radiation of 2-mm Al HVL in a 20 × 20 cm field but close to zero for ultrasoft x rays.

EFFECT ON PERCENTAGE DEPTH DOSE ($D_{1/2}$)

As field size increases, the relative depth dose increases because of backscatter (see above). With soft radiation (HVL < 0.5 mm Al), backscatter is negligible (see Fig. 14) and relative depth doses for field sizes ranging from 20 to 200 cm² show no significant variations. With more penetrating radiation (HVL > 0.5 mm Al), the effect of backscatter on the $D_{1/2}$ in treatment areas ranging from 20 to 200 cm² is significant and must be taken into consideration.

EFFECT ON CUTANEOUS RADIATION REACTIONS

For identical exposures, the intensity of radiation-induced skin reactions varies considerably with the field size (see p. 57). In general, small areas tolerate much higher dosages than do large areas (e.g., a field of 2 cm² can be exposed to a maximum divided dose of 15,000 R without serious sequelae, whereas an area of 4 cm² may tolerate only 8,000 R).

EFFECT ON THE CHOICE OF TSD

When the irradiated area is small (1–5 cm diameter) the TSD should be at least 15 cm; larger areas (>10-cm diameter) require a TSD at least twice the diameter of the field in order to insure uniform irradiation of the entire area (see Fig. 18). With the soft x-ray tubes used in dermatologic radiation therapy, the edges of a field with a diameter half the length of the TSD receive approximately 90% of the dosage received by the center of the field (see Fig. 19).

Cones

As a measure of radiation protection, cones should be used whenever possible. The use of metal cones in soft radiation therapy has the following advantages:

1. The TSD can be adjusted precisely.
2. The area to be irradiated is fixed in place through contact with the cone.
3. The direction of the central beam (away from the gonads) can be controlled.
4. Radiation protection is increased.

Exposure Time

Selection of exposure time depends on the dose rate of the x-ray tube and on the tissue dose desired. The time span required to administer the treat-

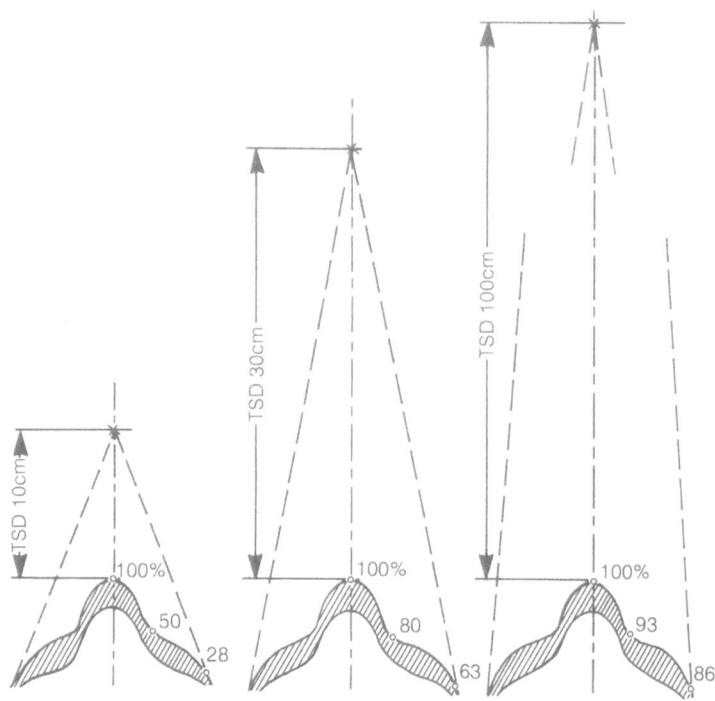

Figure 18. An increase in the TSD reduces variations in incident dose at different points of a curved surface; at the same time, the depth to which the tissue is irradiated uniformly (shaded area) also shows fewer variations with increasing TSD (after Wachsmann 1959).

ment should be long enough to allow accurate measuring by means of the standard timer that is part of the x-ray machine. With a dose rate of about 100 R/min, the doses commonly used in dermatologic radiation therapy can be administered within a few minutes.

Synopsis of the Effects of Changes in Physical Factors

In the past, before accurate calibration methods became available, qualitative effects of varying physical parameters were expressed in a simple formula. Because of significant absorption of longer wavelengths in air it can no longer be used to compute doses for modern x-ray machines, yet it illustrates clearly the basic rule that the intensity of radiation varies directly as the milliamperage and time, and as the square of the kilovoltage, but inversely as the square of the distance.

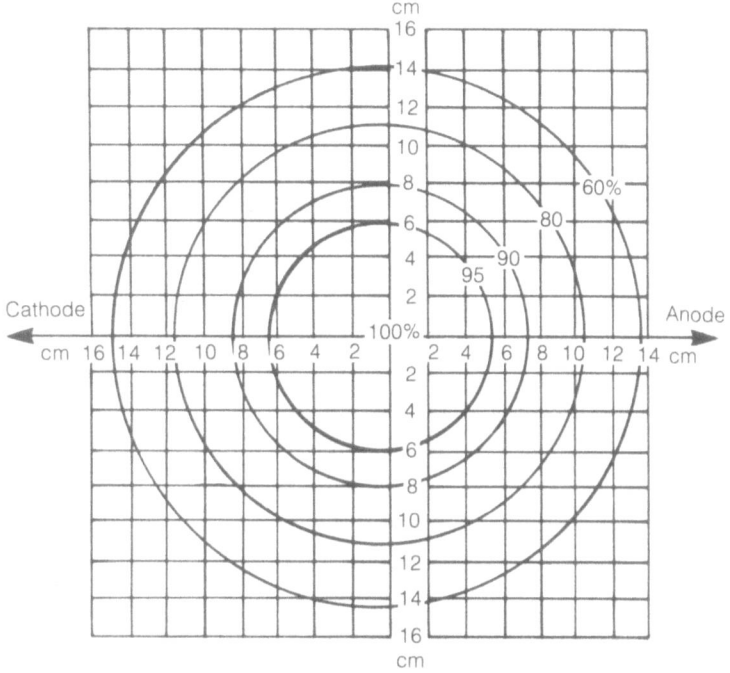

Figure 19. Percentage distribution of dose at TSD 30 cm with a modern beryllium-window tube (Siemens Dermopan).

$$I_{(R/min)} = \frac{mA \times kV^2 \times time}{TSD^2}$$

where *I* equals the intensity of radiation (dose rate in roentgen/minutes), mA the milliamperage, kV the kilovoltage, time the exposure in minutes, and TSD the target–skin distance in centimeters.

The qualitative effects of changing the various physical parameters used in dermatologic radiotherapy are summarized in Table 2 and explained in the following short paragraph (Gorson, in press).

1. The dose rate increases with the increased production of x rays. The number of x rays produced per second depends on the number of the electrons striking the target per second (i.e., the tube current). X-ray production also depends on the energy of the electrons striking the target. The electron energy increases with the tube potential (kilovoltage). Exposure rate also decreases with increasing target skin distance (TSD) because of the inverse square divergence.

TABLE 2

QUALITATIVE EFFECT OF INCREASING PHYSICAL PARAMETERS
USED IN DERMATOLOGIC X-RAY THERAPY

When One Increases (↑):	X-ray tube potential (kV)	X-ray tube current (mA)	Added filter (mm Al)	Target–skin distance (TSD)	Cone size	Exposure time (T)
The quantities listed below will increase (↑), decrease(↓), or remain the same (—) as shown						
1. Exposure rate (R/min) in air	↑	↑	↓	↓	—	—
2. Absorbed dose rate (rads/min) at the skin	↑	↑	↓	↓	↑	—
3. Total skin dose (rads)	↑	↑	↓	↓	↑	↑
4. Effective energy (half-value layer) of the x-ray beam	↑	—	↑	—	—	—
5. The maximum photon energy	↑	—	—	—	—	—
6. The minimum photon wavelength	↓	—	—	—	—	—
7. The backscatter factor	↑	—	↑	—	↑	—
8. Percent depth dose	↑	—	↑	↑	↑	—
9. $D_{1/2}$ value	↑	—	↑	↑	↑	—
10. Surface area in the primary beam	—	—	—	↑	↑	—

SOURCE: Data from Gorson. In Press.

2. The absorbed dose rate is directly proportional to the exposure rate. At the skin, it also increases with the beam size because of increased scatter.

3. The total skin dose depends on the absorbed dose rate and the exposure time.

4. As the tube potential (kilovoltage) is increased, the energy of the electrons striking the tube target increases, thus increasing the average energy of the emitted x rays. Increasing the aluminum filtration selectively absorbs the lower energy (softer) x rays, thus effectively increasing the energy of the transmitted x-ray beam.

5. The maximum photon energy and

6. the minimum photon wavelength depend only on the energy of the striking electrons and hence only on the tube potential (kilovoltage).

7. The backscatter factor increases with photon energy and reaches a maximum around 10-mm Al (0.6-mm Cu) half-value layer, depending on field size. Hence, the back-scattered radiation increases with tube potential (kilovoltage) and with added filtration for the ranges of interest in dermatologic radiation therapy. The backscatter factor also increases with field size.
8. The percent depth dose and
9. the $D_{1/2}$ value increase with photon energy (hence with tube potential and added filtration) because of the greater "penetrating power" of higher-energy x rays. They also increase with target–skin distance (TSD) because of the reduced effectiveness of the inverse square law factor at increasing distances.
10. The surface area in the primary beam increases, of course, with field size or cone size and increases with target–skin distance (TSD) because of the inverse square divergence of the beam.

PRACTICAL ADVANTAGES OF SPECIFYING RADIATION QUALITY IN TERMS OF $D_{1/2}$

1. Selection of physical factors suited to the depth of the lesion is simplified (see Figs. 20 and 21).
2. The dose at the base of the lesion (50% of the surface dose) is easily determined.

Practical Considerations Governing Selection of Treatment Factors

A decisive factor in the selection of treatment conditions is the percentage depth dose of the radiation, which should be varied according to the depth of the lesion (Goldschmidt 1959, 1973, 1976). The goal is nearly uniform irradiation of the lesion.

If radiation quality is:

a. too soft, irradiation of the lesion will not be uniform; the difference between doses at the surface and at the base of the lesion will be too great.
b. too hard, the underlying normal tissue will receive excessive dosage.

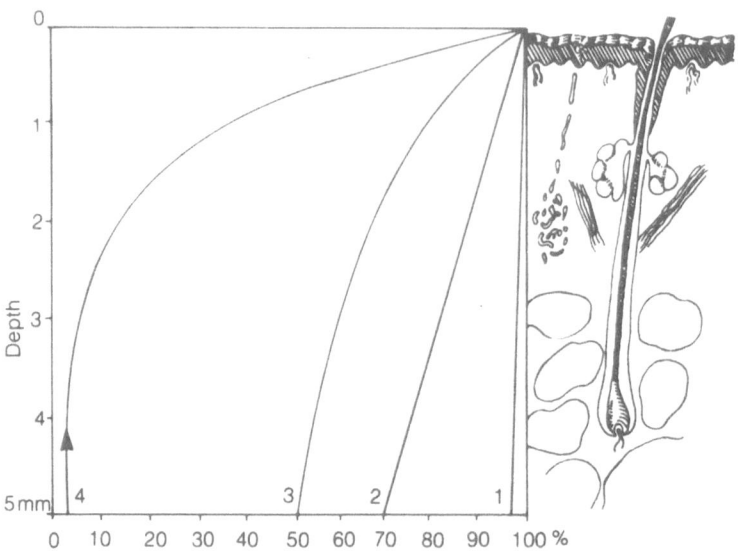

Percentage depth dose

	Type of therapy	kV	mA	Filter	TSD (cm)	Field size (cm²)	HVL (mm Al)
1.	Orthovoltage therapy	122	6	none	30	12.6	3.3
2.	Radium	—	—	0.5 Pt	1	12.6	—
3.	Contact therapy						
	(Chaoul)	60	2	none	5	15.9	2.1
4.	Grenz radiation	10	3	none	36	12.6	0.04

Figure 20. Fall-off of dose in percent of surface dose for various radiation qualities (modified after Reisner 1940 and Ott 1937).

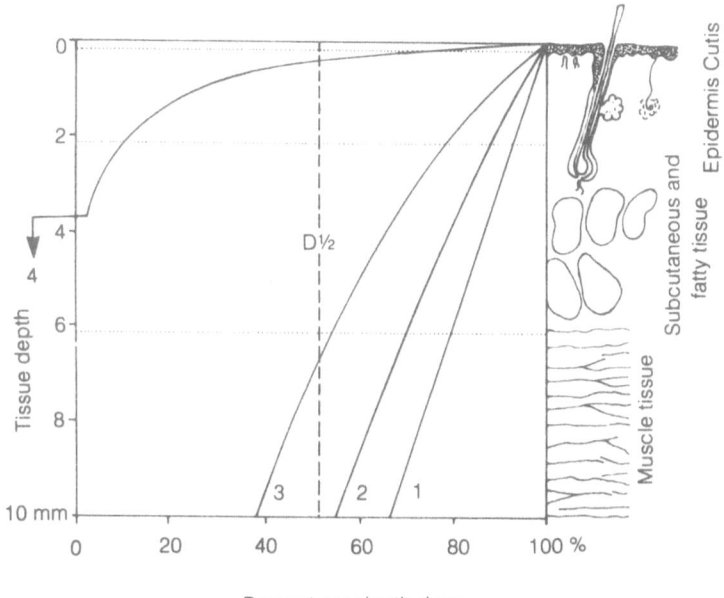

PHYSICAL FACTORS: TSD 30 CM—
FIELD SIZE 100 CM²

	Kilovoltage (kV)	Filter (mm Al)	HVL (mm Al)
1	50	1.2	1.0
2	40	0.9	0.7
3	30	0.6	0.4
4	10	0.05	0.03

Figure 21. Percentage depth dose curves of various radiation qualities and physical factors required to produce these radiations (modified after Holthusen 1959).

TABLE 3

DEPTH OF VARIOUS SKIN LAYERS, SKIN APPENDAGES,

AND IMPORTANT DERMATOSES

I. Normal skin	
Epidermis	0.03– 0.25 mm
Corium	3.0 – 4.0 mm
Hair papilla	2.5 – 3.5 mm
Eccrine sweat glands	2.0 – 3.0 mm
II. Benign dermatoses	
Dermatitis—Eczema	0.8 – 2.1 mm
Psoriasis	0.7 – 3.2 mm
Lichen simplex chron.	1.1 – 4.4 mm
Lichen planus	0.4 – 2.1 mm
Folliculitis, acne	3.0 – 5.0 mm
III. Cutaneous tumors	3.0 –15.0 mm and up

SOURCE: Modified after Zoon and Werz, 1957.

Compromise: the radiation quality should be selected to suit the depth of the pathologic process (Schirren 1959; Wachsmann 1957, 1959, 1970).

> *Rule of Thumb:* The $D_{1/2}$ should closely approximate the depth of the irradiated lesion.

Data indicating the depth of various skin strata and skin appendages and of some of the most important dermatoses are summarized in Table 3.

> *Example:* Irradiation of lichenified hand eczema
> - Depth of lesion: ca. 4 mm
> - $D_{1/2}$: 4 mm
> - Soft x rays: HVL, 0.2 mm Al; TSD, 30 cm
> - Dosage: 3×75 R at weekly intervals.

Combinations (Fig. 20) of physical factors frequently used in dermatologic radiation therapy are summarized in Table 4. The practitioner should consult the tables provided by the manufacturer of his or her therapy unit.

1.9   METHODS OF DERMATOLOGIC RADIOTHERAPY

Grenz-Ray Therapy

Grenz rays are ultrasoft x rays (see p. 8) that are produced by beryllium-window tubes at kilovoltages of 10–20 kV. At the beginning of this century, special grenz-ray tubes with windows made of Lindemann glass (lithium

TABLE 4

PHYSICAL FACTORS REQUIRED TO PRODUCE VARIOUS RADIATION QUALITIES
USED IN DERMATOLOGIC RADIOTHERAPY

Type of radiation	kV	TSD (cm)	Filter (mm Al)	HVL (mm Al)	$D_{1/2}$ (mm)	mA	Dose rate (R/min)
Grenz-ray therapy	10	10	—	0.02	0.25	25	500–1000
	20	10	—	0.03	0.5	25	500–1000
Soft x-ray therapy	30	30	0.3	0.2	4	25	100
	45	30	0.7	0.5	10	25	100
	50	30	1.0	0.8	13	25	100
	50	30	2.0	1.4	18	25	∼50
Contact therapy	50	2	0.2	0.15	3	3	8000
(Philips)	50	3	1.0	0.8	7	3	1500
	100	3	2.5	3.5	35	8	5000
Contact therapy	60	1.5	0.2 Cu	4.3	4	8	2200
(Chaoul)	60	3	0.2 Cu	4.3	8	8	700
	60	5	0.2 Cu	4.3	12	8	300

SOURCE: Data from Wachsmann, 1959.

borate glass) were constructed. Grenz rays can be produced by special grenz-ray machines or by the same x-ray units that are used for soft x-ray therapy (10–50–100 kV).

The HVL of the grenz radiation varies with the tube kilovoltage and the inherent filtration. At about 10 kV, the HVL is approximately 0.02 mm Al; the $D_{1/2}$ is about 0.25 mm. At 20 kV (HVL, 0.03 mm Al) the $D_{1/2}$ is 0.5 mm.

Grenz-ray dosimetry poses special problems because of absorption by the chamber wall and by air.

The dose rates obtained with grenz radiation are high (e.g., at 10 kV, with a 1-mm beryllium filter; TSD, 10 cm; HVL, 0.02 mm Al; $D_{1/2}$, 0.025 mm; tube current, 25 mA; the dose rate is about 1,000 R/min). Preferably, the area to be irradiated should be delimited with lead shields and a cone of the desired TSD should be used.

One of the advantages of grenz-ray therapy is that grenz rays are relatively safe because of their low penetration. However, the method is suitable only for very superficial dermatoses. Table 5 lists technical data of grenz-ray machines sold and serviced in the United States.

Contact Therapy

This method was developed by Chaoul in 1931. A similar method was described by van der Plaats in 1934 (van der Plaats 1939). Both techniques employ specially constructed x-ray tubes designed for extremely

TABLE 5

GRENZ-RAY MACHINES (<20 kV)

Manufacturer	J. J. Stark Equipment Co.	Universal X-ray Products, Inc.
Address	29–28 41st Ave. Long Island City N.Y. 11101	4014 West Grand Ave. Chicago, Ill. 60651
Model	Dermex G	Treatmaster Grenz-ray unit
Window	Beryllium	Beryllium
mA	5–10	5
kV	12–15 (18)	20
HVL range (mm Al)	0.02–0.04	0.02–0.04
$D_{1/2}$ range (mm tissue)	0.2–0.5	0.2–0.5
Cooling method	Air	Air

short treatment distances (1.5–5 cm). The tube kilovoltage used is relatively low (50–60 kV). Other characteristics are low penetration, slight to moderate filtration, steep falloff of dosage, and high dose rate. The radiation dosage is therefore concentrated in the lesion, whereas the underlying normal tissue is minimally affected. The contact method was, for a time, very popular in the treatment of skin cancers. Large tumor doses were fractionated' and intracavitary treatment could be given when necessary. Good results were obtained in the treatment of basal and squamous cell carcinomas; the short exposure time was especially advantageous in the management of strawberry marks in infants.

A distinct disadvantage is the limited field size. Larger areas could be irradiated only by consecutively treating several adjacent fields; this involved the danger of overlapping and excessive exposure.

The $D_{1/2}$ used in contact therapy usually ranges from 4 to 12 mm (see Table 4). The relative depth dose should closely approximate the depth of the lesion.

In tumor therapy, surface doses are given in daily fractions of 300–500 R up to a total of 5,000–10,000 R, or until tumor resolution is obtained.

With the introduction and widespread acceptance of soft x-ray therapy, contact therapy has lost favor. Table 6 lists technical data of contact x-ray machines sold and serviced in the United States.

Soft X-Ray Therapy

Introduction of beryllium-window tubes has opened up the 20–50 kV range for dermatologic radiation therapy (Proppe 1958; Schirren 1959). The low inherent filtration of beryllium (1 mm Be is roughly equivalent to 0.01

TABLE 6

CONTACT X-RAY MACHINES

Manufacturer	Philips
Address	Philips Medical Systems Inc.
	710 Bridgeport Ave.
	P.O. Box 484
	Shelton, Conn. 06484
Model	RT 50
Window	Beryllium
mA	2
kV	10–50
HVL range	0.02–0.7
$D_{1/2}$ range	0.25–4.5 mm
Safety devices	Six standard kV–filter combinations with automatic control
Cooling method	Air

mm Al) permits the passage of soft x rays that are lost if window material with greater inherent filtration is used. The dose rates obtained in this manner are high, allowing short exposure times. It is worth emphasizing that with soft radiation the desired dosage falloff is a result of the radiation quality, whereas with contact radiation (extremely short TSD) it is obtained by divergence of the radiation. (See p. 35 and Fig. 16). A distinct advantage of soft x-ray therapy is the fact that large areas may be irradiated in one sitting, which permits treatment of extensive lesions as a single field.

Most modern x-ray therapy units have built-in safeguards against technical errors (insertion of wrong filter, etc.) and standardized dose rates, using a limited set of kilovoltages in combination with the appropriate filters. These measures have significantly increased the safety of dermatologic radiation therapy.

ADVANTAGES OF SOFT X-RAY THERAPY

1. X rays of low penetration can be utilized therapeutically.
2. Radiation quality can be selected to suit the depth of the lesion (HVL, $D_{1/2}$).
3. High dose rates are obtained, permitting:
   a. short exposure times
   b. greater TSD
   c. irradiation of larger areas
   d. a selection of filter–kilovoltage combinations with the dose rate remaining constant (e.g., 100 R/min)
   e. a choice of radiation qualities optimally suited to various therapeutic objectives.
4. Because of the rapid dosage falloff in the tissue, the radia-

tion dose is largely contained in the pathologic process; damage to the underlying normal tissue is thus kept to a minimum.

(Although the dosage falloff is also very rapid in contact therapy, the mean energy imparted is considerably greater; the ratio of integral doses in soft x-ray therapy and in contact therapy is about 1 : 3. Only fast electrons and beta-ray emitters are, in this regard, superior to soft x radiation.) Table 7 lists technical data of soft x-ray machines sold and serviced in the United States.

Superficial X-Ray Therapy

The superficial (low-voltage, standard, conventional) x-ray technique was the most widely used dermatologic radiation method before the advent of the beryllium-window machine (Cipollaro and Crossland 1967; Walter and Miller 1969). The radiation, employed in the treatment of superficial lesions, was produced by a tube with a Pyrex (glass) window at 60–100 kV with a HVL of 0.7–1.0 mm Al and a TSD of 15–30 cm. Normally, no additional filtration was used. The $D_{1/2}$ of this radiation varies from 7 to 10 mm tissue and is satisfactory for most dermatologic conditions, even though it is more penetrating than necessary, because most dermatoses involve only the upper 3–5 mm of skin. The same treatment units have also been used in "filtered techniques" for deep skin lesions or skin cancers where radiations of 120–140 kV filtered through 3-mm Al with a HVL of 2–3 mm Al were used. The $D_{1/2}$ of this radiation is 20–30 mm; it is indicated only in tumors that are extremely deep and rarely seen in dermatology. Table 8 lists technical data of superficial x-ray machines sold and serviced in the United States.

Intermediate X-Ray Therapy

Treatment of rare pathologic processes extending to a depth of about 3 cm calls for very penetrating radiations. The physical factors required to produce such radiation ($D_{1/2}$ 2–5 cm) are: tube kilovoltage, 80–100–140 kV; HVL, 2–2.5 mm Al; TSD, about 10 cm. Superficial therapy units or deep therapy machines that fulfill these requirements may be used. Rare indications include deep carcinomas, occasional sweat gland abscesses, actinomycosis, etc.

Orthovoltage Therapy

Deep x-ray therapy ($D_{1/2}$ 5–8 cm) has no place in dermatologic therapy; it should be administered exclusively by radiation therapists. Physical factors are 150–400 kV; HVL, 0.8–5 mm Cu.

TABLE 7

Soft X-ray Machines (10–50 or 5–100 kV)

Manufacturer	Bucky X-ray International Inc.	General Electric Co.	Philips Medical Systems Inc.	Siemens Corp.
Address	30 E. 81st Street New York, N.Y. 10028	Medical Systems Div. P.O. Box 414 Milwaukee, Wis. 53201	710 Bridgeport Ave. P.O. Box 484 Shelton, Conn. 06484	186 Wood Ave. South Iselin, N.J. 08830
Model	Dermatological Combination Therapy machine	G.E. Maximar 100	RT 100	Dermopan II
Window	Beryllium	Beryllium	Beryllium	Beryllium
mA	5–10	5	8–10	25
kV	5–100	30–100	10–100	10–50
HVL range (mm Al)	0.02–3.0	0.3–2.0	0.025–2.5	0.02–1.8
$D_{1/2}$ range (mm tissue)	0.2–35	1–30	0.3–30	02.–20
Safety devices	Automatic filter control above and below 15 kV	Color-coded filters, flashing light without filter	Ten standard kV–filter combinations with automatic control	Four standard kV–filter combinations with automatic control
Cooling method	Air	Air	Closed water circulating system	Closed water circulating system

TABLE 8

SUPERFICIAL X-RAY MACHINES (60–120 kV)

Manufacturer	Picker X Ray	Universal X-ray Products, Inc.
Address	2880 Comly Road Philadelphia, Pa. 19154	4014 West Grand Ave. Chicago, Ill. 60651
Model	Zephyr	Treatmaster X-ray unit
Window	Pyrex	Pyrex
mA	5–10	3–5
kV	60–120	60–95
HVL range (mm Al)	0.25–3.0	0.25–3.0
$D_{1/2}$ range (mm tissue)	8–30	8–30
Safety devices	Color-coded filters	Color-coded filters
Cooling method	Air	Air

The various methods of dermatologic radiation therapy and their advantages are summarized in Table 9.

Fast Electrons (Electron Beam Therapy)

Monoenergetic fast electrons, such as those produced by particle accelerators (linear accelerator, betatron), are gaining importance in radiotherapy. They differ from x rays in three essential points that appear to justify the expense and complexity of equipment and procedure:

1. Monoenergetic electrons have a defined depth of penetration in the tissue; beyond that point, the dosage is practically nil.
2. Irradiation of the tissue is virtually uniform in the layer extending to about half the penetration depth of the beam. The point of maximal dosage is reached at about one-third of the depth of penetration.
3. Beyond the uniformly irradiated layer, dosage falloff is very rapid.

Electron beam therapy therefore offers an ideal solution to the problem of avoiding damage to underlying structures. However, dose distribution in the superficial layers is greatly dependent on the field size, because the electrons are subject to considerable lateral scatter on entering the tissue.

The mechanism of action of fast electrons is similar to that of x rays; the relationships between dosage and biologic effectiveness are, however, slightly different.

At present, electron beam therapy is available only in large radiation

TABLE 9

RADIOTHERAPEUTIC METHODS AND APPROPRIATE THERAPY UNITS

Method	kV	HVL (mm Al)	$D_{1/2}$ (mm)
1. Grenz ray therapy	6–20	0.01 –0.1	0.25– 2.0
2. Soft x-ray therapy	20–60	0.1 –1.4	3.0 –18.0
3. Contact therapy	15–60	0.2 –3.5	2.0 –20.0
4. Superficial therapy	60–120	0.6 –2.4	7.0 –40.0
5. Intermediate therapy	80–140	2.0 –2.5	20.0 –50.0
6. Orthovoltage therapy	150–400	0.8 –5.0 Cu	50.0 –80.0

Therapy unit	Advantages	Disadvantages
1. Grenz-ray apparatus	Relatively safe	Suitable only for very superficial dermatoses
2. Soft x-ray therapy unit	Suitable for treatment of all types of dermatoses and cutaneous neoplasms	Special safety measures required
3. Contact therapy unit	Suitable for tumor therapy	Limited TSD and field size
4. Superficial therapy unit (also suitable for intermediate therapy)	Suitable for deeper dermatoses and skin cancers	Special safety measures required
5. Intermediate therapy unit	Deep penetration	Too penetrating for most dermatologic lesions
6. Orthovoltage therapy unit	Very deep penetration	Too penetrating for most dermatologic purposes

centers. Its chief indications are malignant skin tumors (especially near bone and cartilage).

Monoenergetic beta particles (cathode rays) produced in a Van de Graaff generator or a linear accelerator have also been used successfully in the palliative whole body treatment of generalized lymphomas, particularly mycosis fungoides (Fromer et al. 1961). Energies vary from 1 to 4 MeV; at 25 MeV of energy, the average penetration of the electrons is 7 mm of tissue. The depth of penetration of electrons into tissue is proportional to their energy. The adaptation to the depth of the lesion and the very rapid falloff of energy in the underlying structures make electron beam therapy theoretically appealing and well suited for dermatologic purposes. In mycosis fungoides, the recommended dose is 100–200 rads, up to 2,000 rads. Good results have also been reported in Kaposi's sarcoma, reticulum cell lymphoma, and in the cutaneous manifestations of Hodgkin's disease.

1.10 ROENTGEN THERAPY APPARATUS USED IN DERMATOLOGIC RADIATION THERAPY

A complete x-ray unit consists of the following component parts:

1. A source of electrons, furnished by a separate filament circuit which provides low-voltage current to heat the filament of the x-ray tube.
2. An electromotive force to drive the electrons at high speed to the target; this is provided by the high-voltage current.
3. Devices for current control and regulation of variables, such as voltage, amperage, and time.
4. A means of rectification.

Most x-ray generators used in dermatologic radiation therapy employ either two-valve, half-wave rectification or self-rectification. The high voltage produced by the generator as well as the current supplying the cathode is carried to the x-ray tube by means of cables. To increase the scope of the treatment range, the x-ray tube is equipped with a thin but highly resistant beryllium window. The anode is cooled by circulating oil, which in turn is cooled by circulating water or air.

Special filters are provided that serve to change the spectral distribution of the radiation by preferentially absorbing the soft components, thus producing more penetrating radiation. Cones and diaphragms or other collimators are used to restrict the area exposed to the useful beam.

By the use of a fixed set of treatment factors (kilovoltage, filtration, TSD) and constant tube current, the safety of operating x-ray equipment has been increased considerably.

The x-ray machine should be convenient to operate and the radiation source should be easily maneuverable. The patient is usually positioned on a chair or table. Tube housing, control panel, and high-voltage generator are often combined in a compact, mobile unit. An adjustable wall arm has also been found useful.

1.11 RADIONUCLIDES

Only radioisotopes of interest to dermatologists are discussed here. Most dermatologists have abandoned the use of radium because of radiation protection problems.

Gamma-Ray Sources

COBALT-60

Radioactive cobalt (^{60}Co) has a half-life of 5.3 years. It has been used to some extent in dermatology, especially in the treatment of tumors not easily accessible by other methods, e.g., in the auditory canal or the naso-labial fold. Because of the high integral doses involved and radiation protection problems, the use of gamma-ray emitters in dermatotherapy is no longer advocated.

Beta-Ray Emitters

Beta radiation penetrates only a few millimeters into the skin.

PHOSPHORUS-32 (^{32}P)

Phosphorus-32 has a $D_{1/2}$ of 1.2 mm and a half-life of about 14 days.

STRONTIUM-90 (^{90}Sr)

Strontium-90 decays to yttrium (^{90}Y) in a process involving beta emission. The $D_{1/2}$ of ^{90}Sr–^{90}Y is 1.6 mm. Strontium-90 has a half-life of about 20 years, whereas the half-life of ^{90}Y is only 2.6 days. Commercially available ^{90}Sr preparations emit only yttrium electrons; the softer ^{90}Sr beta rays are filtered out with a 0.1-mm nickel filter. Strontium preparations have been used experimentally in very superficial lesions (hemangiomas, basal cell carcinomas, squamous cell epitheliomas). Safety measures must be observed carefully. Hazards are incorporation in bone tissue and long half-life; only sealed applicators should be used.

Alpha-Ray Emitters

THORIUM X

Thorium X is primarily an alpha-ray emitter ($>90\%$), but it also emits gamma rays. It is a natural degradation product of radiothorium and has a half-life of 3.64 days. Alpha rays penetrate only superficial skin layers. In the past, thorium X was used in the treatment of nevus flammeus, Darier's disease, chronic psoriatic lesions, and eczema. This practice has been abandoned because of the hazards associated with the accompanying gamma radiation (Schirren 1962).

2

General radiobiology

2.1 INTRODUCTION

Many new developments in radiotherapy have their origin in radiobiologic research. It is through continued efforts in this field that we are able to test new types of radiation, study cellular kinetics, and find and apply new sensitizers and protective substances. Radiation protection is an important field of technology that has its foundation in general radiobiology (Rajewsky and Pohlit 1959).

2.2 PRIMARY REACTIONS TO PHYSICAL PROCESSES

Whenever ionizing radiation traverses body tissues, it transfers energy to them by the processes of atomic excitation and ionization (see p. 3). Ionization is the mechanism by which the radiation is absorbed; only absorbed energy can be effective in producing biologic reactions. The mode of action by which the absorbed energy produces changes in the living cell has been the subject of a vast amount of research, and a number of theories have been formulated.

Chemical Reactions

WATER

Radiation products of high biologic activity are those produced by activation of water (free H· and OH· radicals, hydrogen peroxide, and other chemically and biochemically active peroxides). Molecular oxygen plays an important part in their formation; the more O_2, the more H_2O_2 (Fritz-Niggli 1959).

PROTEINS

Roentgen rays may alter the configuration of proteins. Sulfhydril groups are a prominent target. The dosage required to cause such changes, however, is several thousand rads.

AMINO ACIDS

Radiation liberates pharmacologically active substances (e.g., histamine-like compounds). However, this occurs only with very high dosage.

NUCLEIC ACIDS

X rays may cause breaks in the chains of the double helix that serves as a template for polymerizing enzymes in DNA and RNA synthesis. It is now generally believed that this type of injury is the basic mechanism by which cellular reactions to radiation are produced (for a literature review, see Streffer 1969).

Biologic Effects of Radiation

The concept of "direct action" implies that biologically important molecules, such as nucleic acids and proteins, are directly affected and altered by ionization and excitation. Radiobiologic effects within the tissue are dependent on the number of ions produced. The target theory postulates that sensitive structures, such as chromosomes, are struck directly by ionizing radiation (Rajewsky and Pohlit 1959). An example of direct action would be gene mutation.

"Indirect action" occurs when radiochemical changes in the environment produce chemical alterations in biologically essential material via toxic intermediate products. The theory of indirect action postulates that a biologic unit undergoes radiation-induced changes when a sensitive target is hit indirectly by energy transferred through free radicals formed in the irradiated material.

GENETIC EFFECTS

Even minute doses of radiation (several rads) may induce irreversible chromosome breaks and aberrations. By chromosomal analysis, such structural chromosome changes can be demonstrated in the peripheral blood of humans exposed to radiation.

Ionizing radiation increases mutation rate as a function of dosage. Mutation rates are also influenced by linear energy transfer (LET) (see p. 48) and spacing of dosage. A dose of 30 rads to the gonads doubles the rate of spontaneous mutation. Because there is no known threshold dose for genetic damage and even minute doses may cause injury, it is imperative in dermatologic radiation therapy to shield the gonads of patients of or below reproductive age (see p. 61).

EFFECTS ON CELLS

Roentgen rays will kill cells directly when given in sufficiently large dosage (more than 10,000 R). Lymphocytes succumb to smaller doses. Cell division is reduced by very small doses of x radiation. In addition to temporary inhibition of mitosis, radiation may cause irreversible suppression of cell proliferation (inactivation). All mammalian cells are inactivated according to identical dose–effect curves (e.g., 200 R inactivate about 50% of the cells; 1,000 R, more than 99% (for a literature review, see Hug and Trott 1970; Trott 1972).

EMBRYONIC DAMAGE

Ionizing radiation may induce malformations in embryonic tissue. The probability of such injury is dependent on the dose (minute doses are sufficient!) and the stage of development. In man, periods of increased radiation sensitivity are the first 2 months following fertilization, until organogenesis is completed. The risk of malformation in humans is significantly increased after exposure to radiation doses as low as 10–20 rads.

CARCINOGENIC EFFECTS

It has been shown in man that the risk of leukemia or other malignant disease increases as a function of dosage. The existence of a threshold dose below which there is no increased risk has not been proved conclusively.

2.3 FACTORS INFLUENCING
THE RESPONSE TO RADIATION

Dose Dependence

The radiation effect is a function of dosage, whether given as a single dose or divided into fractions.

Effect of Oxygen Tension

The injurious effect of ionizing radiation on living tissue increases with the concentration of molecular oxygen within the cell; hypoxia, in contrast, reduces the radiation effect.

The term "oxygen enhancement ratio" (OER) has been introduced as a measure of the oxygen effect. The OER indicates the ratio of radiation doses needed to produce identical effects in oxygen-free and in oxygen-rich cells. For x rays, the OER is 2.5–3.0. The OER, in turn, is a function of the linear energy transfer (LET), which is defined as the rate of energy loss per unit length of path by an ionizing particle traversing a material medium and is expressed in keV/μm.

Radiation with low LET has a high OER; radiation with high LET has a low OER.

Linear Energy Transfer (LET) Dependence

The biologic effectiveness of radiation is dependent on the linear energy transfer (LET) and, therefore, on the type of radiation (see p. 15). In dermatologic radiation therapy it is well to remember that the biologic effects of x-radiation qualities in the 50–200 kV range, and even in the range between 10 and 50 kV, are nearly identical, provided irradiation of the target organ is adequately homogeneous.

Time Dependence

Cells exposed to fractional dosage have the ability to recover from sublethal radiation damage. The effect of fractional irradiation is therefore smaller than that of an equal single dose. Recovery is complete after a maximum of 24 hours.

Biologic and Clinical Factors

Increased blood supply enhances radiosensitivity, whereas impaired circulation (e.g., compression by cones) reduces it (see "Oxygen Effect").

Sensitizers (e.g., actinomycin D) increase radiosensitivity; protective substances (e.g., cysteine) reduce it (for a literature review, see Franke 1972; Wiskemann 1972). In dermatologic practice, these substances are currently of no significant value.

The degree of differentiation and the location of the irradiated tissue are important factors. The inguinal, axillary, and anal regions are more sensitive than the thorax, abdomen, or face. Temperature elevation increases radiosensitivity; so does an increased metabolic rate.

Metabolic diseases, such as diabetes mellitus or gout, increase radiosensitivity of the skin; a similar effect is observed following administration of certain drugs, such as iodine. The patient's constitution and age are important considerations; radiosensitivity decreases with advancing age.

Summary

The biologic radiation effect is seen as a function of dosage, dose distribution, dosage schedule, radiation quality (LET dependence), and oxygen tension.

General biologic factors, such as constitution, localization, type of tissue, age of patient, metabolic disorders, previous administration of certain drugs, degree of sensitivity to radiation, temperature, and blood supply in the irradiated tissue, have a significant influence on the reaction of the skin to radiation.

2.4 ABSORPTION OF X RAYS IN SKIN, SUBCUTANEOUS TISSUE, CARTILAGE, AND BONE

The fundamental law of the biologic action of x rays states that the magnitude of the biologic effect is determined largely by the radiant energy absorbed. Equal biologic effects (independent of the energy of the radiation) occur only when the absorbing biologic tissue has the same energy absorbing properties for various radiation qualities. With radiation in the range below 100 kV, this condition is satisfied when the effective atomic number of the various tissues is the same. Because the effective atomic number of human skin is sufficiently similar to that of air (7.7) and water (7.2), the energy absorbed in the skin per roentgen of exposure is virtually independent of the radiation quality.

In fatty tissue (effective atomic number, 6.0), the biologic effect per roentgen is reduced. Conversely, the absorption in bone is about seven times as great as in water; hence, the biologic effectiveness of soft radiation relative to the exposure measured in roentgens is higher in this type of tissue.

Applied to dermatologic radiotherapy, these observations permit the following conclusions:

1. With regard to the epidermis and the dermis, it is irrelevant whether harder or softer radiation (below 100 kV) is used, as long as the skin is irradiated uniformly.
2. The fatty tissue of the subcutaneous layer absorbs relatively soft radiation at a lower rate than do the epidermis and dermis (about 0.6 times as much).
3. Bone tissue absorbs about six to seven times as much of soft radiation as it does of hard radiation (see Fig. 22). This is of no great consequence in dermatologic radiation therapy because only minimal doses of soft radiation should reach the bone when proper radiation qualities are used.
4. Cartilage absorbs about 1.1–1.5 times as much as the skin.
5. Muscle tissue has the same radiation absorbing properties as the skin (Fig. 22).

2.5 EFFECTS OF X RAYS ON SKIN AND SKIN APPENDAGES

Roentgen Erythema

After a single exposure to conventional x radiation, the skin develops a reaction that proceeds in a rhythmical wavelike pattern. The observations described below are based on the following treatment conditions: 180 kV; filter, 0.5 mm Cu; HVL, 0.9 mm Cu; TSD, 23 cm; surface dose rate, 40 R/min; field size, 6 × 8 cm. With this penetrating radiation, a "standard erythema" is produced by a skin dose of about 800 R, which has been called "skin erythema dose" (SED)—a concept often used in the past as a quantitative measure of the biologic effect of x rays.

The erythematous reaction is composed of the early reaction (early erythema); the main reaction (main erythema), the onset and intensity of which is a function of dosage; and the late reaction (for a schematic representation, see Fig. 23).

1. Early reaction (early erythema). The minimum dose required to produce an early erythematous reaction with hard x rays is about 450 R (i.e., about 60% of the skin erythema

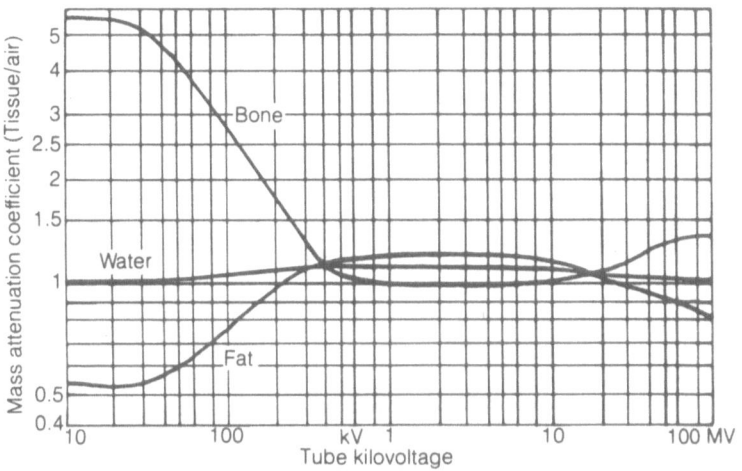

Figure 22. Absorption of conventional x radiation of various energies in water and in tissues (after Wachsmann and Dimotsis 1957).

dose). The reaction may occur immediately or up to 24 hours after irradiation and last for 2–3 days. Subsequent pigmentation is slight.

2. Main reaction (main erythema). The main erythema appears about 8 days after irradiation and increases in intensity during the next 8 days. The intense redness of the skin may be followed by hyperpigmentation. Onset and intensity of the reaction are dependent on dosage.

3. Late reaction (hyperpigmentation). Hyperpigmentation may follow the main erythematous reaction. The transition between the two phases is subject to considerable variation;

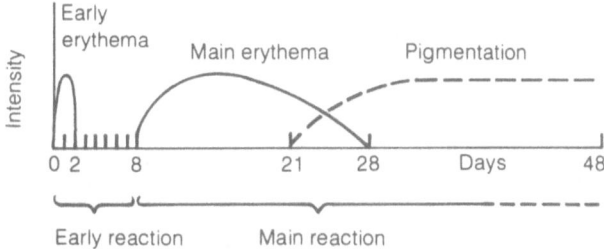

Figure 23. Schematic representation of the erythematous reaction following administration of the "skin erythema dose" (after Flaskamp 1930).

51

as a rule, hyperpigmentation appears after the main erythema has subsided (about 28 days after exposure). It may persist for several years or even for a lifetime. In rare cases, hyperpigmentation may occur without antecedent erythematous reaction.

The tolerance limit of a 6 × 8 cm area of skin for a single radiation dose of hard x rays is about 800 R. With higher doses, the changes are usually not completely reversible but are followed by erosive or ulcerative reactions, which eventually lead to the late sequelae associated with chronic radiodermatitis (atrophy, dryness, alopecia, telangiectasis, induration, hyperpigmentation, hyperkeratosis, etc.).

Fractional administration of the dosage increases the tolerance limit and causes overlapping of the various phases of cutaneous response; erythematous and erosive reactions occur after higher dosages.

Histology of the Cutaneous Reactions to Radiation

In the epidermis, the mitotic rate is reduced during the early erythematous phase; the nuclei show pyknotic and polymorphic changes. At dosages of 900–1,100 R, epitheliolysis and epidermal atrophy may ensue.

In the corium, the wavelike reaction pattern is associated with vasodilation and inflammatory changes. At 100–1,000 R, the smaller vessels show swelling of the endothelial cells, followed by necrosis of the vascular wall and thrombosis.

The elastic and collagen fibers of the corium are fairly resistant to radiation. The effects of x rays on sweat glands, sebaceous glands, and hair follicles are described below.

Effect on Hair Follicles

Exposure of anagen hair roots (matrix and papilla) to a dose of 350–400 R leads to temporary epilation after about 3 weeks. Regrowth starts after 8–9 weeks.

Exposure of the hair follicles (scalp: HVL, 1.45 mm Al; TSD, 25 cm) to a dose of 1,000 R (at least 600–800 R) may produce degenerative changes in the matrix cells of the hair bulbs, resulting in permanent alopecia.

Effects on Sebaceous Glands and Sweat Glands

Sebaceous glands and sweat glands are similar in their radiosensitivity. Temporary functional impairment is seen 5–6 days after administration of about 400 R. Following a single permanent epilation dose (600– 800 R), only a few sebaceous glands persist, and their function and morphology are greatly altered.

In terms of clinical radiotherapy, these observations indicate that irreversible suppression of the skin appendages cannot be achieved without chronic radiation damage to the skin.

Radiodermatitis

The term "radiodermatitis" is used to designate injuries to the skin and mucous membranes following excessive doses of conventional types of radiation. Radiodermatitis may be classified as acute or chronic (Epstein 1962).

ACUTE RADIODERMATITIS

Acute radiodermatitis may occur after routine administration of a high dose of x rays or radium (e.g., to a malignant tumor) or after accidental overexposure. Clinical symptoms are erythema, edema, vesiculation, erosion (see Fig. 24 on p. 55), ulceration, and pain. Acute radiodermatitis may be of the first, second, or third degree, depending on the dosage administered.

FIRST-DEGREE ACUTE RADIODERMATITIS

A first-degree reaction is characterized by erythema or hyperemia with edema. Pruritus may occur. The reaction reaches its maximum in 10–14 days, usually subsides in the third or fourth week. Pigmentation may persist for several weeks or months. Alopecia may be temporary or permanent, depending on the dosage.

SECOND-DEGREE ACUTE RADIODERMATITIS

There is no sharp line of demarcation between first-degree and second-degree radiodermatitis. Intense erythema, edema, vesiculation, erosion, and superficial ulceration are the predominant symptoms (Figs. 24, 34c). The erythema usually develops earlier than that of a first-degree reaction; its color changes from scarlet to purplish red to livid. The epidermis is partially or completely destroyed, leaving an eroded surface. Pain may be severe. Spontaneous healing occurs after 6 weeks to 3 months. There may be permanent alopecia with atrophy or scarring of the skin.

THIRD-DEGREE ACUTE RADIODERMATITIS

Deep ulceration or necrosis is commonly classified as acute radiodermatitis of the third degree (see Fig. 25). In this severe reaction, erythema may develop within 24 hours; the skin becomes livid to brownish red. Edema is pronounced and the epidermis exfoliates. The depth of the reaction depends on the quality and amount of radiation received; it may involve subcutaneous tissue, bone, or cartilage. The irradiated area undergoes progressive necrosis, ulceration, or dry gangrene. The surrounding tissue shows intense inflammation and pain is severe. The ulcer shows little tendency to granulate and healing is very slow. In some instances, repair may proceed steadily after a delay of several months. An ulcer that has not healed within 12–18 months may undergo malignant changes.

Under favorable conditions, third-degree radiodermatitis may heal with scar formation.

COMPLICATIONS

Complications of exudative or ulcerative radiodermatitis include secondary bacterial infections and malignant degeneration.

CHRONIC RADIODERMATITIS

Chronic radiodermatitis (see Fig. 26a and b) may develop immediately following an acute reaction, or its onset may be delayed for several years or even decades. Repeated exposure to small radiation doses over long periods of time also may lead to chronic radiodermatitis; it is frequently seen in professional groups (physicians, dentists, x-ray technicians, etc.) as a result of occupational exposure without adequate protection.

The chief clinical symptoms are atrophy (either wrinkling or "hidebound skin"), teleangiectasis, sclerosis, pigmentary changes, hyperkeratosis, ulceration, and malignant changes. Atrophy of the sweat glands and sebaceous glands, resulting in dry and shiny skin, and dystrophy of the nails may occur.

These late sequelae may be aggravated further by mechanical, thermal, or chemical irritants (see p. 56).

Chronic radiodermatitis occurs most frequently after x irradiation but is also seen following administration of radioactive cobalt or radium. Chronic radiodermatitis caused by excessive doses of grenz radiation or thorium X is usually more superficial and benign, although the tendency to pigmentary changes is often annoying. Malignant degeneration is an exceedingly rare complication of chronic radiodermatitis secondary to grenz-ray therapy.

TREATMENT OF RADIODERMATITIS

In the treatment of skin cancer, dermatologic radiotherapy may produce a first- or second-degree acute radiodermatitis that is therapeutically desirable

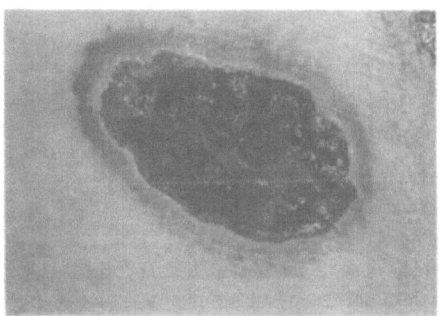

Figure 24. Erosive reaction 12 days after conclusion of treatment of a skin cancer (single fractions of 200–350 R daily, total dose 5,350 R; HVL, 0.3 mm Al; TSD 30 cm).

and may even be used as a guide in determining the required dosage. In the opinion of many experts, a malignant neoplasm should be irradiated until an "erosive reaction" associated with tumor involution is obtained. When treating radiodermatitis, the physician must differentiate between the acute and the chronic type.

TREATMENT OF ACUTE RADIODERMATITIS

Treatment of acute radiodermatitis is very similar to that of other types of acute dermatitis. Erythematous reactions may be treated with powders or lotions, whereas erosions are best treated with antibiotic creams. Steroids added to antibiotic ointments or creams will reduce inflammation. In rare instances, analgesics or sedatives may be indicated.

TREATMENT OF CHRONIC RADIODERMATITIS

Patients with chronic radiodermatitis should be kept under long-term medical supervision to insure adequate care of the injured skin and detection of early malignant changes. The use of mechanical and chemical irritants (i.e., scrubbing with soaps, detergents) and exposure to actinic and thermal agents should be reduced to a minimum. The affected areas should be kept lubricated. Pigmentary changes may be concealed with Covermark or similar preparations. Keratoses should be either excised or treated by electrocoagulation and curettage. Necrotic tissue may be removed with proteolytic enzymes. Because secondary infections may aggravate chronic ulceration, they should be treated promptly with antibiotic ointments.

Indolent ulcers or other late third-degree reactions that show delayed healing (see p. 54) should be treated surgically as soon as possible, because conservative measures require months or even years of treatment, with no assurance of success. Excision and plastic repair are advised.

Teleangiectasia may be controlled by electrocoagulation.

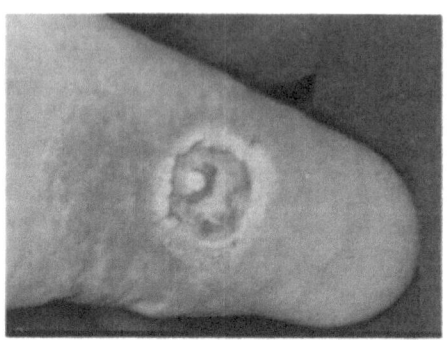

Figure 25. Acute radiodermatitis, third degree (radiation ulcer) following radiotherapy of a malignant melanoma with massive doses.

AGGRAVATION OF RADIODERMATITIS BY SECONDARY FACTORS

Ulcers may develop in radiation-damaged areas showing the classic signs of chronic radiodermatitis: atrophy, sclerosis, teleangiectasia, and pigmentary changes (for details see p. 54). Ulceration may be caused by the atrophy and reduced reparative powers of the radiation-injured tissue or by secondary external factors, such as mechanical, chemical, or actinic irritation. Secondary internal factors contributing to the development of late sequelae are diabetes mellitus, peripheral circulatory disorders, or hepatic impairment.

Differential diagnosis should rule out a recurrence of the tumor. However, aggravation of radiodermatitis by secondary factors is suggested when development of the ulcer is rapid, complicated by secondary bacterial infection, and limited to a portion of the irradiated area. Severe pain is another suggestive feature. Because the clinical picture of a radiation ulcer often resembles that of a recurrent carcinoma, the diagnosis may have to be established histologically.

TREATMENT OF RADIODERMATITIS AGGRAVATED BY SECONDARY FACTORS

A therapeutic trial should be made before a biopsy is taken. However, if treatment is not successful within 6 weeks, this course should be abandoned.

Antibiotic ointments with or without corticosteroids have been found effective in the management of late sequelae (see p. 55); significant improvement may be obtained within a few days, and the lesion may heal completely within a short time. If healing is delayed or complicated, surgical excision and repair are indicated. Prophylaxis includes restriction of mechanical, chemical, actinic, and thermal irritants.

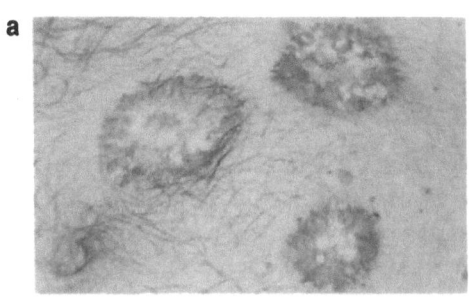

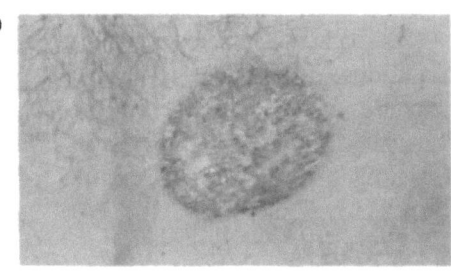

Figure 26. a. and **b.** Chronic radio-dermatitis (trunk). Marked telan-giectasia.

If there is any suspicion of tumor recurrence (no improvement after 6 weeks of treatment), a biopsy is strongly indicated.

Influence of Physical Treatment Factors on Cutaneous Reactions to Radiation

DOSAGE

The reaction of the skin to radiation depends primarily on the dose administered, i.e., on the energy absorbed.

RELATIVE DEPTH DOSE

The intensity of the biologic reaction to radiation is also greatly dependent on the size (or depth) of the irradiated volume, which in turn is a function of radiation quality, field size, and TSD. In terms of clinical radiotherapy, this means that following irradiation of a larger volume (hard radiation, large field) a longer recovery period is required than after treatment of a smaller volume. (For example, a 2-cm^2 area of skin exposed to 15,000 R in fractional doses and a 4-cm^2 area exposed to 8,000 R will require the same time to recover from the exudative reaction.)

> *Rule of Thumb:* Small areas tolerate considerably higher doses than do large areas.

The effect of the TSD on the percentage depth dose in soft radiation therapy is insignificant (see p. 23).

RADIATION QUALITY

Ionizing radiations produced in the conventional range of 10–200 kV cause radiodermatitis when administered in sufficient doses, regardless of radiation quality; only the depth of the reaction is affected by the quality of the rays. The shorter the wavelength, the deeper is the damage to the skin and underlying structures (see also "Percentage Depth Dose Curves," p. 25).

Grenz rays are less damaging to the vascular layers because of the rapid dose falloff; therefore the erythema dose (surface dose required to produce roentgen erythema) for extremely soft grenz rays (10 kV) is very high (about 2,500 R). Even large doses of grenz rays do not produce epilation (see also Figs. 20 and 21).

Hard radiations (HVL, ca. 1 mm Cu) impart a uniform dosage to deeper skin layers (10 mm).

With soft radiations (HVL, 0.4 mm Al), dose falloff in the tissue is fairly rapid, so that at a depth of 6–7 mm only 50% of the incident dose is received (see Fig. 21). With very hard radiations (>200 kV), the erythema dose is higher than with hard radiation, because the mean ionization density decreases beyond 200 kV.

The erythema dose as a function of radiation quality is shown in Fig. 27.

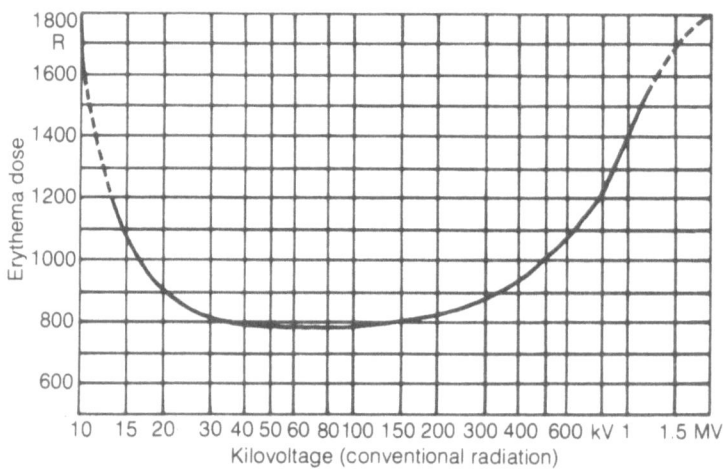

Figure 27. Erythema dose (mean values) as a function of radiation quality (after Wachsmann and Dimotsis 1957).

A single dose of fast electrons also produces a wavelike reaction pattern in the skin. In the energy range between 1.5 and 3.5 MeV, however, the intensity of the cutaneous reactions is about one-third greater than after x irradiation.

TIME–DOSE RELATIONSHIP

In addition to the relative depth dose and radiation quality, the timing of radiation treatment has a significant influence on its effect. In this context, the principles of protraction and fractionation deserve a brief discussion.

PROTRACTION

Protracted treatment means prolongation of exposure time at a reduced dose rate (e.g., a dose of 500 R may be administered in a few minutes, or it may be spread out over 10 minutes). Tissue tolerance is increased slightly by protraction of the dosage; however, with modern soft x-ray machines adjustable to dose rates of 20–5,000 R/min, protraction is considered impractical and insufficiently advantageous.

FRACTIONATION

Fractionation means subdivision of the dosage into small fractions, a technique that—like protraction—increases tissue tolerance. This is illustrated by the following example: with hard radiation, a dose of 800 R is required to produce a standard skin erythema at a dose rate of 40 R/min. By dividing this dosage into fractions given at 24-hour intervals, it is possible to administer a considerably higher total dose (e.g., 4×320 R $= 1,280$ R or 12×160 R $= 1,920$ R) and obtain the same degree of skin erythema (Rajewski and Pohlit 1959). Fractionation therefore spares the vascular connective tissue of normal skin and increases the selectivity of the radiation. Normal cells recover faster than tumor cells after each fractional dose; at the end of the treatment series normal cells can still recover whereas tumor cells are no longer able to do so.

The individual fractions usually range from 200 to 600 R for malignant skin tumors, with 24-hour intervals between treatments. The relationship between different individual doses, total accumulated dose, and overall treatment time of various carcinomas has been studied by Strandqvist, Paterson, and Friedman (see Johns and Cunningham 1969). For benign disorders, the fractions are generally lower (25–100 R), and intervals of more than 24 hours are not uncommon (e.g., in antiinflammatory radiotherapy). Intervals ranging from 1 week to several months may be indicated in the treatment of benign tumors (e.g., hemangiomas, keloids).

3

Radiation
safety and protection

3.1 GENERAL CONSIDERATIONS

The following recommendations are summarized from the radiation protection guide published by the American Academy of Dermatology. The reader is also referred to the detailed discussion of radiation protection and shielding in Cipollaro and Crossland (1967), and Gladstein (in press).

The first step in minimizing the hazards of radiation is to avoid unnecessary exposure of patients by using nonradiative therapeutic measures that will do the job as well. Second, when radiation therapy is necessary, it is important to select a quality of radiation properly suited to the depth of the pathologic process, a quality penetrating enough to reach its base but not so penetrating as to damage deeper structures. The third step is the protection of the patient's radiation-sensitive tissues, such as the lenses of the eyes, the thyroid gland, the gonads, and the blood-forming organs. Noncutaneous adverse sequelae of excessive and/or improper radiation therapy (e.g., cataracts, thyroid tumors, hematologic disorders) are discussed in detail by Rudolph and Goldschmidt (in press). In modern dermatologic radiotherapy, they can be prevented completely.

3.2 SHIELDING

Protection against the useful beam is usually obtained by using a cone and/or lead shield the aperture of which sharply restricts the area to be exposed. The recommended thicknesses of lead for shields are given in Table 10. These are the thicknesses of lead that reduce the useful beam to 5% of its original value.

The shielding ability of lead rubber, lead vinyl, and other materials may be expressed in terms of "lead equivalent." This term denotes the thickness of lead affording the same attenuation.

The therapist can minimize exposure of the patient to scattered and leakage radiation during dermatologic radiation therapy by:

1. Using cones that confine the beam to the area to be treated
2. Directing the beam away from the gonads
3. Placing lead shielding on the treatment table
4. Placing lead shielding over the patient's body, particularly from the umbilicus to the knees.

The gonadal doses received with and without these protective procedures have been measured by several dermatologists; they showed that the gonadal dose is greatly reduced when these precautions are taken. For example, when the face was exposed to 100 R the gonadal dose was reduced from 105 mR (milliroentgens) to 6 mR by 0.5 mm of lead shielding placed on the treatment table and over the patient's body.

Techniques

FACE

When diffuse eruptions of the face are treated, the scalp, eyebrows, ears, lips, and neck are shielded with lead or lead rubber plastic cut to fit the

TABLE 10

LEAD PROTECTION FOR DIFFERENT
QUALITIES OF RADIATION

Tube potential (kV)	HVL (mm)	Lead (mm)
60[a]	1.2 Al	0.10
100	1.0 Al	0.15
100	2.0 Al	0.25
100	3.0 Al	0.35
140	0.5 Cu	0.7

SOURCE: National Bureau of Standards *Handbook*, No. 76.
[a] The radiation produced at 60 kV is filtered in order to give a half-value layer of 1.2 mm of aluminum. Although the useful beam has a higher HVL than that produced at 100 kV, the hardest rays produced at 60 kV are not as hard as those produced at 100 kV; therefore, less lead is required to reduce the useful beam to 5% of its original value.

patient. A lead rubber plastic shield or apron is placed over the patient's body, particularly from the umbilicus to the knees. Shielding materials with a lead equivalent of 0.5 mm of lead are practical for most superficial dermatologic x-ray therapy techniques (see Table 5). With the patient lying in a supine position, the head is placed on a pillow in order to direct the useful beam away from the gonads (see Fig. 28).

NECK

When the neck is irradiated, particular attention must be given to protection of the thyroid gland. If soft radiations, such as grenz rays, are used, the dose to the thyroid gland is exceedingly small. However, if more penetrating rays are required, close shielding will reduce the depth dose to the thyroid gland. During irradiation of the posterior aspect of the neck, the use of a cone and lead shields furnishes adequate protection for the scalp.

CHEST

In the treatment of widespread dermatoses, the use of large cones is preferred. Care should be taken to avoid overlapping exposures. When cones cannot be used in rare instances, two exposures may be necessary. Each focal point falls about 5 cm below the midclavicle. These two focal points

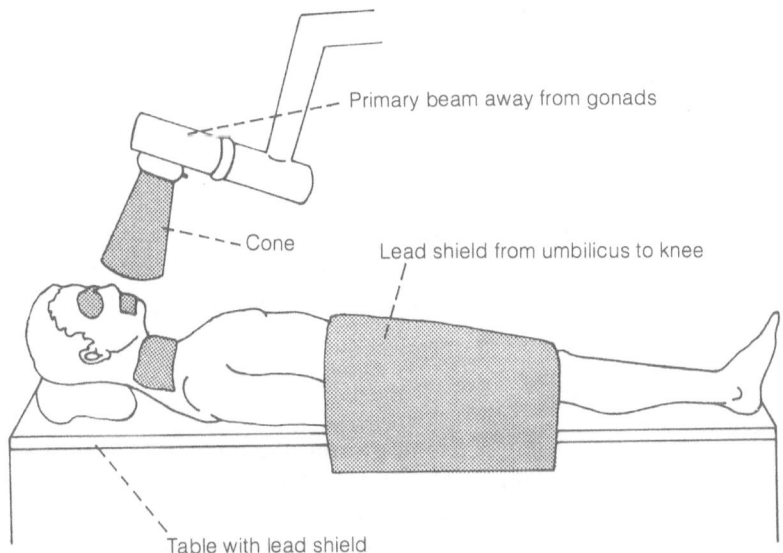

Figure 28. Radiation protection measures for radiotherapy of facial region (from Goldschmidt 1973).

should be at least 30 cm apart. Lead shielding protects the neck, head, and gonads.

BACK

Diffuse eruptions of the back may be treated with large cones or by selecting three focal points, one in each midscapular region and a third at the level of the tenth to twelfth thoracic vertebrae. Lead shields are used to cover the neck and head as well as the pelvic area.

AXILLA

In the treatment of the axilla, the patient lies in a supine position. A cone is used and the beam is directed away from the gonads. A lead shield placed over the pelvic area reduces the gonadal dose. Shielding of the thyroid area is advisable.

PELVIC AREA

Whenever it is necessary to give radiation treatment to any part of the body between the umbilicus and the knees or sacral area of a person of either sex from birth up to the end of the reproductive age, the softest quality of radiation that can be effective is used. If a harder quality of radiation is necessary, the use of cones and a thickness of lead shielding greater than that used for other areas of the body gives more protection to the gonads. Directing the useful beam away from the gonads further reduces the gonadal dose.

SOLES

The soles are best treated by placing the patient on the x-ray table in a prone position with the feet propped up on pillows so that the plantar surfaces are facing the ceiling. To reduce gonadal exposure, the x-ray beam is directed perpendicularly. A lead shield is placed over the sacral area and the upper portions of the thighs to protect the gonads from leakage radiation.

UPPER EXTREMITIES

When treating the hand, forearm, or arm, the therapist can provide excellent protection by seating the patient so that the side of his or her body is against the table. If lead rubber is not permanently attached to the table, a sheet of it is placed under the part to be treated. A sandbag placed under the hand allows the primary beam to be directed away from the gonads. Lead rubber over the forearm and arm protects the body from scattered and leakage radiation. During irradiation of the forearm, the wrist rests on a sandbag and the arm is covered with lead rubber. The extensor surface of the arm can be treated with the patient leaning forward so that his or her shoulder rests on the edge of the table. The flexor surface of the arm can be treated with the patient leaning backward in his or her chair, or placed in a supine position, with his or her arm extended over the edge of the table.

3.3 DOSE LIMITS

Occupational Exposure

Recommended dose limits (also known as maximum permissible doses) have been published by various radiation protection agencies (see Tables 11 and 12). They are usually expressed in rem, the "dose equivalent", based on the concept of relative biologic effectiveness (RBE) which is reserved for radiation protection purposes (see p. 15). It should be emphasized that the exposure of patients for medical and dental purposes is not included in these dose limits.

Maximum Permissible Cumulative Dosage for Benign Dermatoses

In the treatment of skin cancers, acute local skin reactions and secondary, chronic, late radiation sequelae (telangiectases, atrophy, fibrosis, pigment changes) are considered unavoidable and acceptable to a certain degree as a small penalty for the elimination of a malignant tumor. In the treatment of benign skin conditions, however, acute and chronic radiation reactions are totally unacceptable. Uncertainty as to the total permissible radiation dose that can be given safely to any skin area per lifetime has been eliminated by the monumental catamnestic study by Sulzberger et al. (1952) at the New York Skin and Cancer Unit.

After examining 1,500 of 2,907 patients who had been given low-voltage superficial x-ray therapy 5–23 years previously, they found no evidence that fractional superficial roentgen ray treatments given in weekly doses of 75–85 R up to a total of 1,000 R predisposed to malignant alteration. Total doses of up to 1,000 R produced no cosmetically disturbing side effects. In only one out of 87 patients who had received fractional doses between 1,000 and 2,000 R mild nonmalignant sequelae (dryness and slight mottling) were noticed. On the basis of these studies, the authors proposed a maximum of 1,000 R in fractional doses as a safe upper limit

TABLE 11

DOSE LIMITING RECOMMENDATIONS OF

NATIONAL COUNCIL ON RADIATION PROTECTON (NCRP)

Type of exposure	Dose (rems per year)
Occupational exposure	
Combined whole body	
Prospective annual limit	5
Retrospective annual limit	10–15
Long-term accumulation	$(N - 18 \times 5)$[a]
Skin	15
Hands	75 (25/qtr)
Forearms	30 (10/qtr)
Other organs, tissues, and organ systems	15 (5/qtr)
Pregnant women	0.5[b]
Public, or occasionally exposed individuals	0.5
Occasionally exposed medical students	0.1
Population	
Genetic	0.17
Somatic	0.17
Emergency	
Life saving	
Whole body (older than 45 years)	100
Hands and forearms	200
Total	$\overline{300}$[c]
Less urgent	
Whole body	25
Hands and forearms	75
Total	$\overline{100}$[c]
Family member of radioactive patients	
Under age 45	0.5
Over age 45	5

SOURCE: "Basic Radiation Protection Criteria," NCRP Report No. 39, National Council on Radiation Protection and Measurements, 7910 Woodmont Avenue, Washington, D.C. 20014.
[a] Where N is age in years.
[b] Rems per gestation period.
[c] Dose limit at time of emergency.

of radiation. Pillsbury (1961) considers this dosage an absolute maximum and suggests never to exceed a total divided dose of 500 R in view of the potential additive effect of actinic damage in light-exposed areas. Domonkos (1971) limits fractional x-ray treatments to a total of 800 R. It should

TABLE 12

SUMMARY OF DOSE LIMITS FOR INDIVIDUALS AS RECOMMENDED BY THE
INTERNATIONAL COMMISSION ON RADIOLOGICAL PROTECTION (ICRP)
(REMS PER YEAR)

Organ or tissue	Adults occupationally exposed	Members of the public
Gonads, red bone-marrow	5	0.5
Skin, bone, thyroid	30	3[a]
Hands and forearms; feet and ankles	75	7.5
Other single organs	15	1.5[b]

SOURCE: "Protection Against Ionizing Radiation From External Sources," ICRP Publ. 15. Pergamon Press, Oxford, 1970.

[a] 1.5 rems in a year to the thyroid of children up to 16 years of age.

[b] In any 1 year the maximum permissible doses should not be exceeded, but in a period of a quarter of a year up to one-half of the annual MPD may be accumulated. If necessary, the quarterly quota may be received as a single dose, but the Commission believes that it would be undesirable for doses of this magnitude to be repeated at close intervals.

be emphasized in this context that skin cancers resulting from x-ray therapy are seen almost without exception in patients who in years past have had massive doses of x rays that have far exceeded the total doses now recognized as safe. In most instances, these excessive doses were caused either by inadequate calibration techniques or by a lack of understanding of cumulative radiation effects, which became general knowledge only after 1930.

It is advisable to observe the maximum cumulative dosage limit of 1,000 R (5,000 R for grenz rays) in all benign skin conditions, whereas common skin cancers and other malignant and premalignant conditions, such as Kaposi's sarcoma, Bowen's disease, lentigo maligna, mycosis fungoides, and Hodgkin's disease, are exempt from these limitations.

4

Radiotherapy
of cutaneous tumors

4.1 GENERAL CONSIDERATIONS

Indications for X-Ray Therapy of Cutaneous Tumors

In the treatment of benign tumors, selection of a suitable therapeutic modality is often determined by cosmetic considerations. In the case of malignant tumors, however, the method of choice is the one with the highest therapeutic effectiveness (Keining and Braun-Falco 1970). With the exception of special indications for surgical or chemosurgical treatment, radiation therapy is particularly advantageous in the management of skin cancers exceeding 1 cm in diameter. This is especially true of cutaneous neoplasms in the facial area, where surgical measures may cause severe disfigurement. Because surgical removal of tumors involving nose, lips, and eyelids is often followed by considerable scarring, x-ray therapy may be given preference in these cases, provided the dosage can be kept at an acceptable level (Goldschmidt 1975). The appearance of radiation sequelae is dependent to a considerable degree on localization; the skin of the trunk, for example, is more sensitive than the facial skin. Selection of appropriate dosage is dependent on a variety of factors: type of tumor, field size, and especially the time factor (fractionation). The therapist must establish an optimal time–dose relationship that takes into account the total dosage required to destroy a malignant tumor as well as the healing tendency of the surrounding tissue (see Johns and Cunningham 1969). Fractional dosage is always preferable to intensive therapy.

Advantages and Disadvantages of Radiotherapy

Compared to other therapeutic methods, radiotherapy has the following advantages (Baer and Kopf 1965; Kopf 1971):

1. No additional tissue defect is created because only the tumor tissue is destroyed. In certain crucial areas, such as eyelids and tip of the nose, avoidance of damage to surrounding normal tissue is an especially desirable feature of radiation therapy.
2. A sufficiently large field of irradiation insures that the x-ray treatment also destroys malignant tissue that is not clinically apparent. In general, a safety margin of 5–10 mm from the visible border of the tumor (e.g., basal cell or squamous cell carcinoma) to the perimeter of the irradiated field is recommended.
3. Dermatologic x-ray therapy causes less emotional aggravation than surgical treatment, especially in elderly patients.
4. The method is painless, with the exception of slight discomfort during the period of acute erosive radiodermatitis.
5. In most cases, patients can continue to work during x-ray therapy; hospitalization is rarely necessary.
6. Additional therapeutic measures, such as plastic surgery, are usually not required.
7. Vital organs (e.g., eyes) can be effectively protected during radiation therapy of the orbital region.
8. Radiation therapy of skin tumors usually does not significantly impair the general condition of the patient.
9. In contrast to surgery, x-ray therapy can be administered regardless of the patient's medication (e.g., anticoagulants) or allergies (e.g., to anesthetics).

Many skin cancers (e.g., basal cell and squamous cell carcinomas) of more than 1 cm in diameter are suitable for dermatologic x-ray therapy (Du Mesnil de Rochemont 1958; Scherer 1967).

Radiation therapy should be used only with caution in the following cases:

1. Malignant tumors measuring more than 8–10 cm in diameter.
2. Malignancies that are in close contact with bone or cartilage (e.g., dorsa of hands and feet) and have invaded the underlying tissue.

3. Malignancies in young patients, especially in the genital area. Youth is a relative contraindication.

Minor inconveniences and discomforts caused by dermatologic radiation therapy, such as alopecia, susceptibility to irritation of the irradiated area, cosmetically annoying radiation sequelae (especially in the trunk area), hypersensitivity to climatic changes, and the necessity of frequent office visits, are not considered serious contraindications to radiotherapy. These disadvantages can be avoided or reduced to a minimum by adequate treatment planning, dosage appropriate to the tumor site, and symptomatic local treatment of the irradiated area.

Sequelae and complications of radiation therapy of skin tumors (usually avoidable with appropriate precautions) are the following:

1. Radiation ulcers, either spontaneous or posttraumatic, may occur months or years after irradiation (cf. "Aggravation of Radiodermatitis by Secondary Factors," p. 56).
2. Painful ulcerations (third-degree acute radiodermatitis, Fig. 25 on p. 56) may appear immediately after irradiation of particularly susceptible areas (such as dorsal aspects of hands or feet); in severe cases surgical repair may be required. With few exceptions, these areas should not be irradiated.
3. Chronic radiodermatitis (Fig. 26 a, b, on p. 57) may develop years or decades after treatment (p. 54). Characteristic findings are atrophy with loss of cutaneous appendages, pigmentary changes, and telangiectases. More severe sequelae (radiation ulcers, premalignant changes, or carcinomas) are rarely encountered in modern dermatologic radiotherapy.
4. Delayed involution of the tumor despite adequate x-ray dosage may occur with certain types of basal cell carcinoma. Histologic examination is inconclusive in these cases, for tumor cells that are still histologically demonstrable at this point may have lost their viability and may eventually succumb. It is therefore advisable to wait 6–9 months before classifying a tumor as radioresistant—provided, of course, that the tumor is not growing and that an adequate dosage has been delivered under appropriate conditions.
5. Conjunctival leukoplakia may occur following irradiation of eyelid carcinomas (Schirren 1959; Kopf 1971). Histologically, this is a benign keratotic reaction with a tendency to heal spontaneously.

71

6. Pseudorecidives are a rare complication of x-ray therapy, starting several months after successful treatment of a tumor. Clinically, the lesions may present as excessive proliferation of granulation tissue, annular hypertrophic scars, or verrucous papillomatous growths. They have a predilection for the face, particularly the nasal region. Histologically, there is hyperkeratosis and acanthosis, with round cell infiltration in the papillomatous epidermis, sometimes with giant cells and vasodilation.

   Contributing factors may be secondary radiation emitted by the metal cone, pressure of the cone on the skin, circulatory disorders, seborrheic skin, age of patient, and type of tumor.

   No treatment is required, but regular checkups are indicated. The lesions generally disappear 2–6 months after conclusion of the treatment. The patient should be advised of the benign nature of these growths; biopsies may be indicated in some cases. Histologic examination is mandatory if the lesions continue to grow or have not disappeared after 6 months.
7. Comedo reactions may occur at the periphery of the irradiated field after treatment, particularly on the nose and cheeks. This reaction may occur after contact therapy as well as after soft x-ray treatment. It usually subsides after several months.

Practical Procedure of X-Ray Therapy of Cutaneous Malignancies

PLANNING OF TREATMENT

DETAILED MEDICAL HISTORY

A detailed medical history (especially of previous radiation therapy) and careful clinical examination (sketches or photographs may be helpful) is essential.

HISTOLOGIC EXAMINATION

Histologic examination of a biopsy specimen from the tumor is necessary. Radiation therapy should never be instituted without previous microscopic examination. Even the seemingly simple clinical diagnosis of a basal cell carcinoma has been found to be erroneous in 10–15% of the cases.

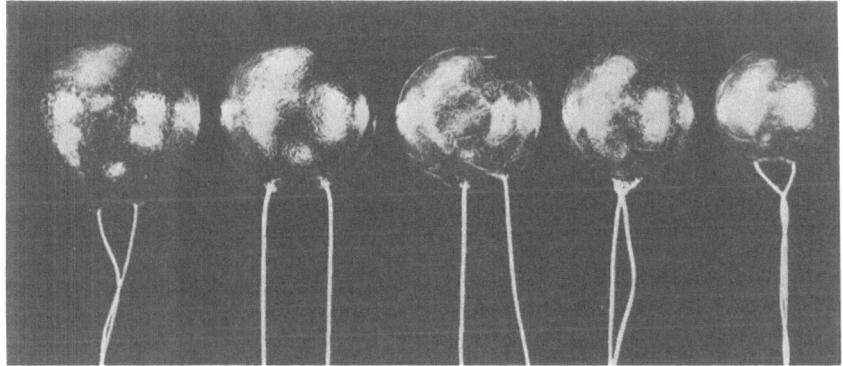

Figure 29. Cup-shaped lead shields for radiation protection of eyeballs. String facilitates insertion and removal (after Knierer and Schirren 1953).

FIELD SIZE (see p. 26)

The size of the irradiated field is often underestimated. The field should be outlined on the skin with a marker, allowing a safety margin of 5–10 mm around the visible perimeter of the malignant tumor. If the field cannot be delimited adequately with a circular cone, a lead shield of 0.5–1 mm thickness may be used to outline the treatment area (Fig. 33 b on p. 85). The diameter of the cone should always exceed the largest diameter of the cutout in the shield. Thyroid gland and gonads must be protected with shields of lead or lead rubber (see "Radiation Protection," p. 62). During irradiation of thin tissues (e.g., eyelids, ala nasi, lips, or ears) additional shielding is necessary to prevent undesirable effects of the exit dose. Figs. 29 to 31 show the technique of shielding the eyes during irradiation of the eyelids (see also p. 63). In rare instances, large tumors with serpiginous or very irregular borders can be separated from the surrounding normal tissue with a 2-mm thick layer of barium sulfate paste. Beyond this margin, lead rubber shields may be used for additional protection.

RADIATION QUALITY

In order to define the quality of radiation, the physical term half-value layer (HVL; see p. 10) has been used for decades. In dermatologic practice, the biologic term "half-value depth" ($D_{1/2}$) has won general acceptance (see p. 21). Physical data for various dermatologic radiation methods are shown in Tables 4 and 9. Optimal results can be expected only if the estimated depth of the tumor is equal to the $D_{1/2}$ of the radiation selected for treatment (Fig. 32) (Goldschmidt 1968). It would now

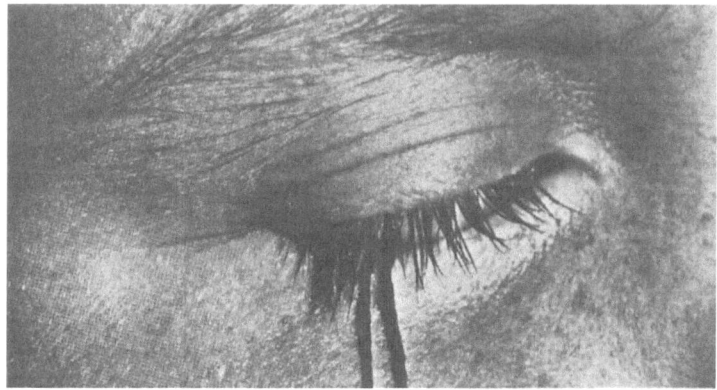

Figure 30. Lead shield inserted into conjunctival sac. String rests on lower lid (from Schirren 1959).

be considered unwise, for example, to irradiate a cutaneous carcinoma limited to superficial skin layers with radiation qualities used for deep therapy ($D_{1/2}$ up to 80 mm). Physical treatment factors commonly used in dermatologic radiation therapy (kilovoltage, filtration, HVL, and $D_{1/2}$) are given in Table 4. Actual depths of cutaneous cancers were reported by Atkinson (1962).

DOSAGE AND MODE OF ADMINISTRATION

For definition of radiation units and other dosimetric concepts see

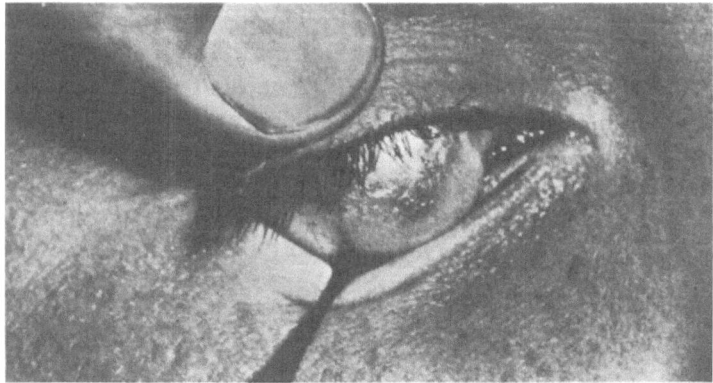

Figure 31. Removal of lead shield by pulling string (from Schirren 1959).

p. 13. In the following paragraphs, dosages are given in roentgens as surface doses (air or incident dose multiplied by backscatter factor). Total dosage is determined by the individual pathologic process; the doses given below should be understood only as guidelines. In addition to radiation quality, spacing of the doses has a significant influence on the therapeutic effect. Protracted and fractional dosage and selectivity are discussed in detail on p. 59; single-dosage "intensive" treatment is discussed on p. 78.

SELECTION OF SUITABLE RADIOTHERAPEUTIC METHODS

The estimated depth of the lesion is the most important factor in selecting a suitable method of irradiation, because the tumor depth should closely approximate the $D_{1/2}$ of the radiation quality used. In addition, the surface area of the tumor has to be considered. The following radiotherapeutic methods are available.

Grenz-ray therapy. This method, which is described in detail on p. 34, can be used only for the treatment of epidermal lesions extending no more than 1–2 mm in depth because the intensity of x rays produced at low voltage (10–20 kV) decreases rapidly within the tissue. Multiple superficial basal cell epitheliomas are often suitable for grenz-ray therapy. The proper dosage should be selected with great care. Dosage schedules for ultrasoft x rays are usually higher than for superficial x rays (Hollander, 1968). Very large single doses ($>1,000$ R) and excessive total doses may result in superficial atrophy even when grenz rays are used.

Because of the possible higher voltages of the soft x-ray tube, soft radiation therapy is preferable in the treatment of flat tumors requiring higher single doses (e.g., lentigo maligna).

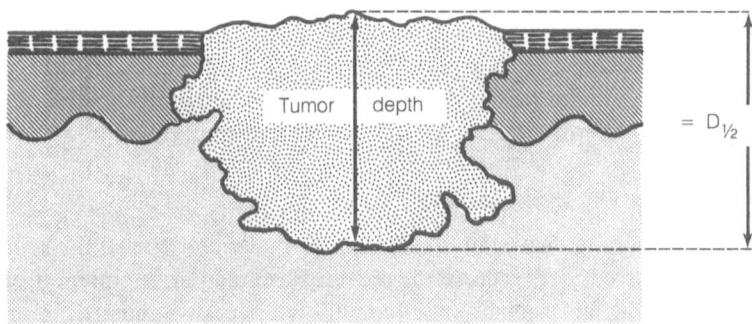

Figure 32. The D$\frac{1}{2}$ of the radiation should equal the estimated depth of the lesion.

Soft x-ray therapy. In recent years, this technique (details on p. 36) has played an increasingly important role in dermatoradiotherapy (Schirren 1959; Goldschmidt 1967). Unlike contact therapy, soft radiation treatment can be used for cutaneous tumors in all layers of the skin, regardless of field size. Other advantages of this method are described in detail on p. 37.

Total dosage of soft x rays in the treatment of malignant skin tumors may vary from 4,000 to 10,000 R, depending on the response (erosive reaction, tumor involution). The individual dose fractions range from 300 to 650 R.

Contact therapy. For definition, characteristics, physical and technical data, as well as apparatus see p. 35.

Daily single doses of 300–1,000 R, up to a total dose of 6,000–10,000 R, have been recommended for the treatment of skin cancers (Domonkos 1965).

Superficial x-ray therapy. Unfiltered low-voltage x-ray therapy with pyrex window machines is eminently useful in the treatment of deeper skin cancers (Cipollaro and Crossland 1967). The $D_{1/2}$ starts at 7 mm and the lowest HVL is 0.6 mm Al. Fractionated doses of 400–800 R are usually given up to a total of 4,000–6,000 R. Filtered superficial x-ray therapy (with 1–2 mm added aluminum filter) yields radiation that is too penetrating for most skin cancers (HVL, 2–3 mm Al; $D_{1/2}$, 12–20 mm).

Intermediate therapy. Physical factors required to produce x radiation for half-deep therapy are given in Table 9. Single doses of 200–300 R up to a total dose of 3,000–5,000 R may be administered, with field sizes ranging from 6 × 8 to 8 × 10 cm. This radiotherapeutic method is indicated only for very deep tumors.

Orthovoltage (deep x-ray) therapy. This method (details p. 38) belongs in the realm of the radiotherapist; it is not useful in the treatment of cutaneous tumors in view of its deep penetration ($D_{1/2}$, 5–8 cm).

EVALUATION OF THE RESULTS

Malignant tumors, with the exception of malignant melanomas, may be considered cured if no recurrence is seen 5 years after completion of treatment. In malignant melanomas, the follow-up period must be more than 5 years. Recurrences are most frequent during the first 6 months after irradiation. Follow-up examination includes inspection and palpation of the irradiated field and regional lymph nodes; distant metastases should also be ruled out.

4.2 RADIOTHERAPY OF MALIGNANT EPITHELIAL TUMORS OF THE SKIN

Among the malignant epithelial skin tumors, basal cell carcinoma and squamous cell carcinoma are predominant. Next to surgical methods, x-ray therapy is the most effective method of treatment for skin cancer. It is important to distinguish between basal cell and squamous cell carcinoma because the latter sometimes requires a larger total dosage. A number of other factors must be evaluated carefully before the proper method of treatment can be selected.

General Considerations

Before radiotherapy can be administered, the clinical diagnosis must be confirmed histologically. Prognosis and treatment planning are greatly influenced by such factors as histologic type of tumor (e.g., sclerodermiform or cystic basal cell carcinoma), degree of differentiation, mitotic rate, stromal reaction in the surrounding area, and the presence or absence of tumor cells in the bloodstream or lymph vessels.

The degree of radiosensitivity is largely dependent on the type of tumor cells involved. For example, lymphoma cells are generally more radiosensitive than tumor cells arising from muscle or bone tissue.

The mitotic rate is another valuable clue: The shorter the cell cycle, the higher the degree of radiosensitivity.

The degree of differentiation of tumor cells is also related to their radiosensitivity. Undifferentiated, biologically immature cells are the most radiosensitive. The following order of decreasing radiosensitivity has been established for cutaneous tumors suitable for radiotherapy:

> Lymphomas
> Basal cell carcinomas
> Squamous cell carcinomas
> Endotheliomas
> Adenocarcinomas
> Sarcomas
> Malignant melanomas

Treatment Planning

The guidelines given on p. 78 should be used to determine field size, radiation quality, TSD, dosage, radiation protection, and shielding.

77

FIELD SIZE

The importance of an adequate field size has been discussed in detail on p. 73. A sufficiently large margin of normal skin (at least 0.5–1.0 cm) is mandatory to prevent peripheral recurrences.

RADIATION QUALITY

Soft x rays are suitable for all types of cutaneous carcinoma.

TARGET–SKIN DISTANCE (TSD)

In most modern x-ray machines, the TSD is standardized (see p. 26). In order to insure sufficiently uniform irradiation of the lesion, the TSD must be in proportion to the size of the tumor and the irradiated field. When curved surfaces are treated, longer target–skin distances are preferable (see p. 26).

DOSAGE AND FRACTIONATION

There is no hard and fast rule as to the total dosage, which should be adapted for each individual case. Fractional doses are always preferable. In general, single doses of 400–650 R are given daily (or every other day); for extensive tumors, the single dose should be smaller (200–300 R) (see p. 27). Total dosage depends on field size, clinical evidence of tumor involution, erosive reaction, and individual radiation doses administered. A standardized method for treating skin cancer was evaluated by Barth et al. (1968) and Kopf (1971). They used 100 kV, 5–10 mA, 0.9 mm HVL, 5 doses of 680 R per treatment, with 2 to 3 day intervals.

SIZE OF TUMOR

In treatment planning, a distinction between "small" and "large" tumors is helpful.

SMALL TUMORS

Small tumors are those not exceeding 4 cm in diameter.

Tumors up to 1 cm in diameter. With field sizes up to 1 cm in diameter, use of the single-dose (massive) technique may be justified in very exceptional cases. A single dose of 2,000–3,000 R of a suitable radiation quality may be administered. If exudative reaction and tumor involution have not occurred after 2–4 weeks, the same dose may be repeated. We prefer fractional dosage, which also yields better cosmetic results.

Tumors up to 2 cm in diameter. Massive single-dose therapy is definitely not advisable in these cases. Larger individual doses (500–800 R) may be given at longer intervals (two times a week). The total dosage may be relatively low (3,500–5,000 R) (Storck *et al.*, 1972; Kopf, 1971).

Tumors exceeding 2 cm in diameter.   Daily treatments are required. Administration of 400–650 R at daily intervals, up to a total of 4,000–8,000 R, is recommended.

Insufficient dosage must be avoided in order to prevent recurrences.

When very prominent tumors are treated, radiation therapy may be interrupted for 8–10 days after a total dose of 3,000–4,000 R, in order to assess the rate of tumor involution. In some cases, electrosurgical planing of markedly raised tumors prior to radiotherapy is advisable to allow the use of softer radiation qualities.

The total dosage obviously also depends on the individual dose: the greater the single dose, the smaller the total dose, and vice versa.

LARGE TUMORS

Large tumors are those exceeding 4 cm in diameter.

Radiation quality.   This is dependent on the estimated depth of the tumor.

Dosage.   Tumors exceeding 4 cm in diameter should be treated with lower single doses (200–350 R) than small tumors. Lesions larger than 10–15 cm in diameter usually are unsuitable for radiation therapy. Total dosage again depends on individual doses and field size, as well as on the rate of tumor involution and the underlying tissue. Total doses of 3,500–6,000 R are usually sufficient. After administering half the total dose, suspend treatment for 1 week to observe tumor regression.

The advantages of soft x rays over contact irradiation are especially evident in the case of large tumors. Soft x-ray techniques can be adapted easily for this purpose; multiple overlapping fields (as in the grid technique of contact therapy) are not required.

RADIATION PROTECTION AND SHIELDING

In patients of reproductive age, the gonads should be shielded with lead (or lead rubber) (see p. 62). The central beam should be directed away from the gonads (Fig. 28). When irradiating a tumor near the gonads, do not expose the gonads to direct radiation; whenever possible, tumors in the anogenital area should be treated by other therapeutic measures. Even when the tumor is located some distance away from the gonads, these may be reached by relatively high doses of radiation when proper shielding is neglected (Witten 1957; Fritz-Niggli 1959; Lorenz 1961).

During irradiation of tumors in areas with underlying bone and cartilage such as the ala nasi or ear, a lead shield should be placed in the nostril or behind the ear. Because the rate of energy absorption is increased in bone and cartilage, tumors in those areas should be treated with smaller doses and a lower $D_{1/2}$. In adults, bone tissue covered only by a thin cutaneous layer may develop trophic changes (e.g., bone necrosis following irradiation of large tumors on the skull). Painful postirradiation chondritis of the ear cartilage may be prevented by selecting a lower radiation quality and smaller fractions (e.g., an exophytic carcinoma of the helix may be treated with radiation having a $D_{1/2}$ of 7–8 mm, administered in fractions of only 400 R). When tumors in the orbital area are treated, the lens must be shielded with eye cups (for details, see p. 73; Figs. 29–31).

Shielding of the surrounding normal skin with lead shields cut to size has also been discussed on p. 73.

Specific Indications

BASAL CELL CARCINOMA

Among the malignant epithelial skin tumors, basal cell cancers present the most frequent indication for soft x-ray therapy. Metastases are exceedingly rare. In radiotherapy two types are differentiated:

- *Superficial basal cell cancer.* This type usually occurs in multiple lesions on the trunk.
- *Infiltrating basal cell cancer.* Nodular basal cell cancer, noduloulcerative basal cell cancer (ulcus rodens), cystic basal cell cancer, morphea-like basal cell cancer, premalignant fibroepithelial tumor (Pinkus). The diagnosis must be confirmed histologically before radiation therapy is instituted.

Radiation quality. The $D_{1/2}$ should equal the depth of the lesion. Very superficial tumors, such as multiple superficial basal cell carcinoma of the trunk, may be treated with grenz rays (4 $\times$ 2,000 R, administered in daily fractions).

Dosage. For general guidelines, see p. 78. Inadequate dosage may lead to recurrences.

Therapeutic results. Rates of cure between 95 and 100% have been reported (Freeman and Knox 1964) (Fig. 34 a, b). In morphea-like basal cell cancer, the success rate is somewhat lower. Deep carcinoma terebrans also has a less favorable prognosis; it is better treated by combined surgical and radiotherapeutic methods or by chemosurgery. Supervoltage radiation or betatron therapy may be indicated in rare cases.

METATYPICAL EPITHELIOMAS

Mixed or intermediate epitheliomas are treated according to the guidelines given for squamous cell cancer and basal cell cancer. In some cases, the total dosage may exceed the usual limits. Irradiation should be continued until an erosive reaction is obtained.

BASAL CELL NEVUS SYNDROME

This hereditary disorder is characterized by multiple brownish tumors located predominantly on the trunk, face, neck, and in the periauricular area and is often associated with cystic bone changes (jaw cysts) and other defects. In the active growing stage, tumors respond well to radiotherapy. Because of the late sequelae that such treatment undoubtedly entails in younger patients, surgical measures are usually preferred.

SQUAMOUS CELL CARCINOMAS

Squamous cell carcinomas frequently occur between the ages of 60 and 80 years. About 90% of all squamous cell carcinomas are located in areas chronically exposed to sunlight (face, head, and dorsa of the hands). Chronic degenerative or inflammatory changes of the skin, as well as scarring and atrophy, are other predisposing factors (e.g., chronic lupus erythematosus lesions, stasis ulcers of long standing, old fistulas, lichen planus of the mucous membranes of long duration, syphilitic glossitis, balanitis xerotica obliterans, and kraurosis vulvae). Long and repeated exposure to chemical carcinogens (e.g., tar, soot) is another etiologic factor. These squamous cell carcinomas, as well as those involving mucocutaneous junctions, have a greater tendency to metastasize to the regional lymph nodes and, later, to internal organs than the more common type arising from solar keratoses. The prognosis is dependent on localization, degree of differentiation, and size of the tumor. Carcinomas of the tongue, vulva, and penis have a relatively poor prognosis, as do anaplastic carcinomas and those exceeding 3 cm in diameter.

Indication. The general considerations discussed earlier (see p. 69) should govern the selection of treatment. Location, size, and degree of differentiation determine whether surgery, radiotherapy, or a combination of both should be used. In the presence of metastases in regional lymph nodes, surgical excision, possibly combined with radiotherapy (orthovoltage or cobalt) ought to be considered.

Radiation quality. The $D_{1/2}$ should equal the estimated depth of the tumor. Soft x rays having a $D_{1/2}$ of 4–8 mm are usually adequate (HVL,

0.2–1.4 mm Al; TSD, 15–30 cm). Very large, ulcerated squamous cell carcinomas may require other forms of ionizing radiation (cobalt-60, electron beam, etc.). Because of their sharply limited range of penetration, fast electrons (betatron therapy, see p. 40) have been found especially effective in the treatment of tumors close to bone and cartilage, e.g., on the dorsa of hands and feet, where routine radiotherapy should be used only with great caution.

Dosage. For general considerations regarding dosage and fractionation, see p. 78. In most cases, individual and total doses are similar to those used in the treatment of basal cell cancer (p. 80). Occasionally, the doses required to obtain an erosive reaction and tumor involution may be slightly larger than those needed for basal cell cancers. Tumors located near bone and cartilage should be treated with lower single and total doses in order to avoid late sequelae, necrosis, or contractures.

Therapeutic results. The effectiveness of radiotherapy is largely dependent on size, site, degree of differentation, and the presence or absence of metastasis at the start of therapy. Cures have been reported in 85% of cutaneous squamous cell cancers measuring up to 3 cm in diameter. Carcinomas of the tongue, the vulva, and the penis respond less favorably to radiotherapy.

Recurrence. Recurrence of squamous cell cancers and basal cell cancers after radiotherapy is usually caused by an inadequacy in field size, $D_{1/2}$, or total dosage.

CARCINOMAS ARISING IN CHRONICALLY DAMAGED SKIN

Atrophic skin has a tendency to develop carcinoma. Chronic degenerative and chronic inflammatory changes also may give rise to squamous cell cancers (see p. 81).

Indication. Radiobiologic considerations favor surgical measures over radiotherapy in the management of tumors developing in chronically damaged skin areas. If a special situation calls for radiotherapy, lower doses, subdivided into small fractions, should be used. Inadequate total dosage must be avoided, however, or recurrence results. Cooperation with a radiotherapist may be advisable. In some cases, electron beam therapy may be preferable.

Therapeutic results. After careful consideration of the risks involved, radiotherapy may yield satisfactory results in selected cases.

Variations of Technique in Different Anatomic Sites

SCALP

Because skin cancers of the scalp are in close proximity to bone and brain tissue, increased absorption of x rays and increased backscatter have to be taken into consideration.

Radiation quality. X-ray qualities should be softer than in other areas of the integument. When the tumor is movable and x-ray films show no evidence of bone involvement, relatively soft x rays (HVL, 0.2–0.4 mm Al; TSD, 15–30 cm; $D_{1/2}$, 3–8 mm) should be administered. If the tumor has infiltrated the underlying bone tissue, electron beam therapy may be considered. In case of extensive bone involvement, surgical measures should be discussed with a neurosurgeon.

Dosage. Fractional doses should be low and treatment should be suspended from time to time. The total dosage may also be relatively low (e.g., 4,800 R, given in fractions of 300 R; $D_{1/2}$, 4 mm). Special care is necessary to avoid complete denudation of the skull with subsequent aseptic bone necrosis, secondary infection, or failure of the wound to re-epithelialize. Even more caution is indicated when large areas are irradiated.

FOREHEAD AND TEMPLE

The same principles apply as in the treatment of the scalp. Caution is indicated because of the close proximity of osseous structures. Following the erosive reaction, reepithelization usually proceeds at a faster rate than in the scalp area.

CHEEK

Because of the thick underlying tissue, irradiation of tumors of the cheek usually presents no special problems. Potential radiation effects on parotid gland and facial nerve have to be carefully considered. Tumors situated in the zygomatic area may require diagnostic x-ray films to rule out bone involvement. When tumors near the mouth are irradiated, the gums should be protected by insertion of a lead shield (0.5-mm thick), covered with a rubber finger cot.

NOSE

Carcinomas of the nose are a good indication for radiotherapy (Goldschmidt 1976) (Figs. 33 a–d on p. 85). Because of the proximity of bone and cartilage, conditions for irradiation are similar to those in the scalp area. In large cancers, irradiation of curved surfaces (see p. 28) may create special problems. A longer TSD avoids an undesirable rapid decrease of radiation intensity in the border of the field. Controlling the direction of the beam is also easier when a TSD of 30 cm is used. Cross-fire techniques or treatment of several overlapping contiguous fields are best avoided.

Deep carcinomas of the nasal area should be evaluated by an ENT specialist and the depth of the tumor should be assessed by diagnostic x-ray examination. The septum and the opposite surface of the mucosa should be protected by placing a rubber-covered lead shield in one or both nostrils.

Radiation quality. Whenever possible, the $D_{1/2}$ should be kept lower than usual (HVL, 0.2–0.5 mm Al; TSD, 15–30 cm; $D_{1/2}$, 3–4 mm). If the growth has invaded cartilage and bone, treatment with harder radiation qualities by a radiotherapist may be required, or other treatment methods may be indicated (chemosurgery or surgery).

Dosage. In large or complicated tumors, fractional doses should be lower than usual (e.g., 300 R at daily intervals).

Therapeutic results. In uncomplicated cases, radiotherapy of carcinomas of the nose yields highly satisfactory results. Scarring is usually less obvious than following surgical methods. Recurrences after radiotherapy are more common with deeply invasive tumors. In this case therapeutic alternatives (surgical excision, chemosurgery, cryosurgery, electron beam therapy, etc.) should be evaluated for each individual case. Deep basal cell cancers of the nasolabial fold also recur more frequently (often because of inadequate field size), particularly when the selected $D_{1/2}$ is not deep enough for this special anatomic region.

EAR

Indication. If the tumor has invaded the cartilage, surgical measures are indicated. Smaller tumors may be treated effectively with x rays, especially in older patients where surgical treatments are more problematic.

Radiation quality. Soft x rays are preferred. A small rubber shield should be placed on the posterior surface of the ear (see p. 79). Recommended treatment factors are: HVL, 0.2–0.4 mm Al; TSD, 15–30 cm; $D_{1/2}$, 3–8 mm.

Dosage. Fractional doses should be kept small (300 R). Because of the proximity of cartilage, treatment should be suspended for about 10 days after 10–12 days of therapy. This minimizes the danger of perichondritis.

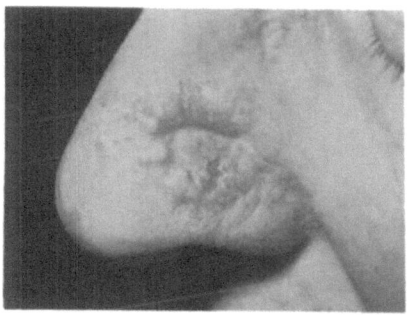

a

Figure 33. a. Large basal cell cancer of the nose of a 75-year old male patient. Recurrence following surgical excision and grafting eight years ago. **b.** Shielding of patient before radiotherapy. **c.** Acute exudative radiodermatitis 2 weeks after last exposure. **d.** Good cosmetic result after radiotherapy with 5,600 R in 500 R fractions. $D_{1/2}$ 13 mm; HVL 0.75 mm Al. Previous graft area still recognizable (from Goldschmidt 1975).

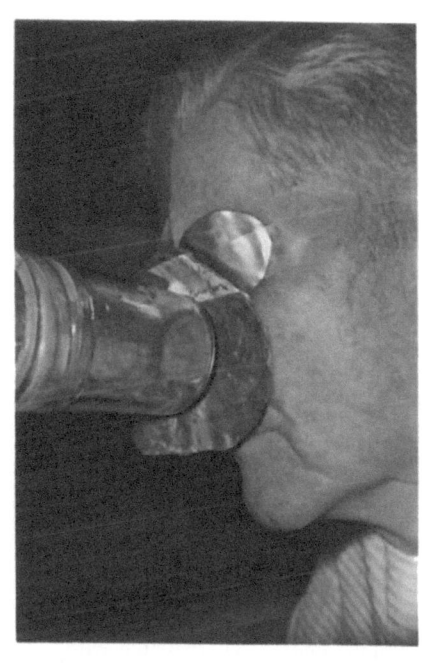

b

c

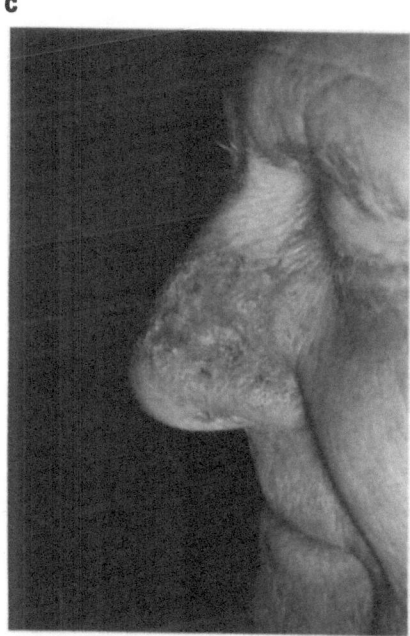

d

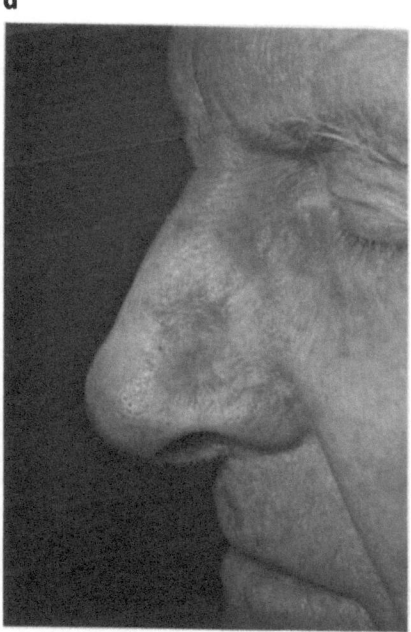

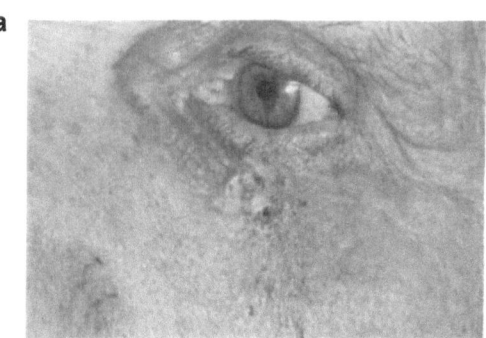

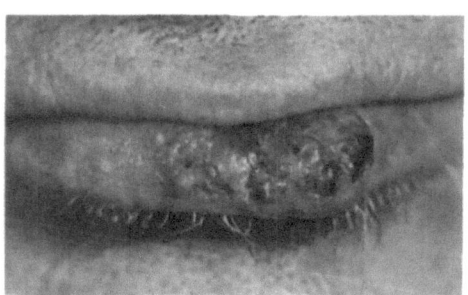

Figure 34. a. Basal cell carcinoma of the lower lid. b. Six months later, after treatment with soft x rays (individual fractions of 500 R daily, total dose 6,500 R; HVL, 0.6 mm Al; TSD 15 cm).

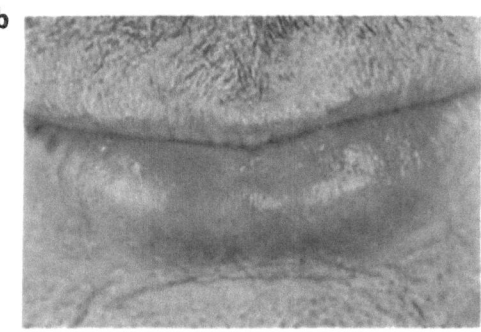

Figure 35. a. Squamous cell carcinoma of the lower lip. b. Five months later, after treatment with soft x rays (individual fractions of 500 R daily, total dose 6,000 R; HVL, 0.9 mm Al; TSD 15 cm).

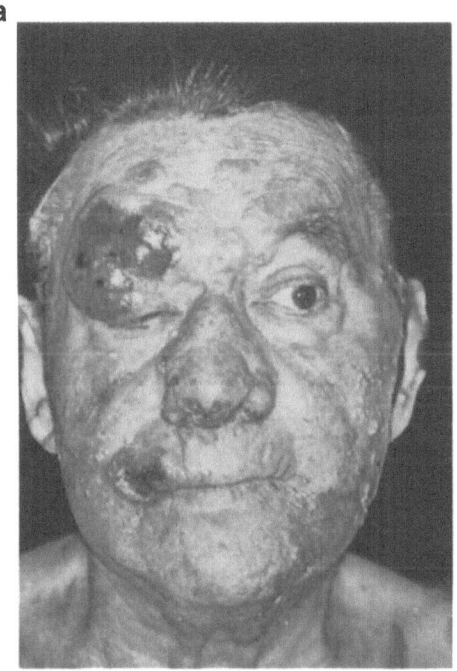

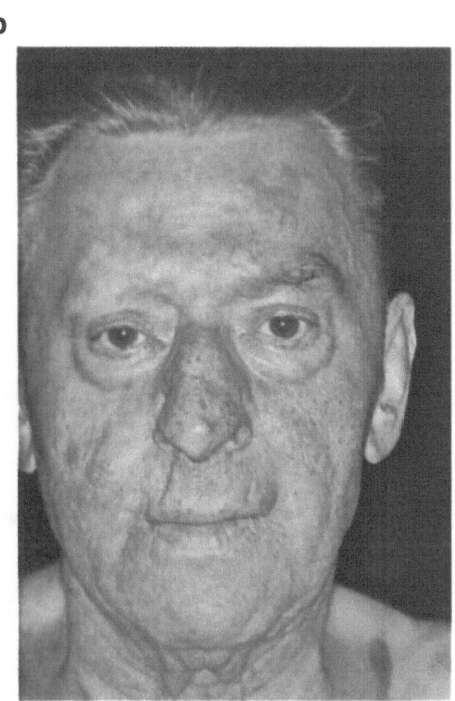

Figure 36. a. Mycosis fungoides.
b. After treatment with soft x rays
(individual fractions of 200 R at
2-day intervals, total dose 1,200 R;
HVL, 0.9 mm Al; TSD 30 cm).

87

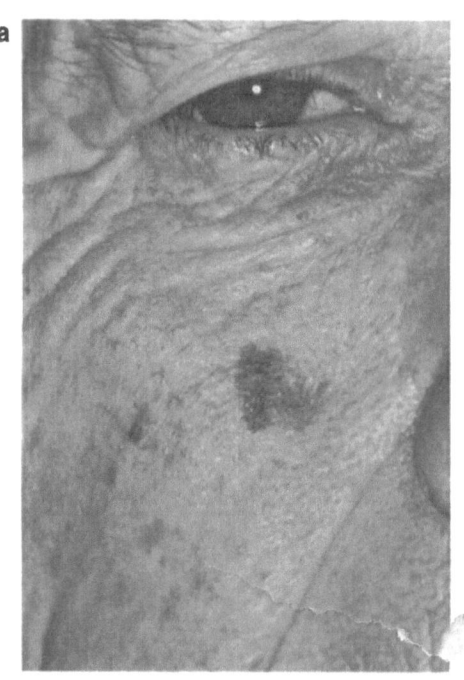

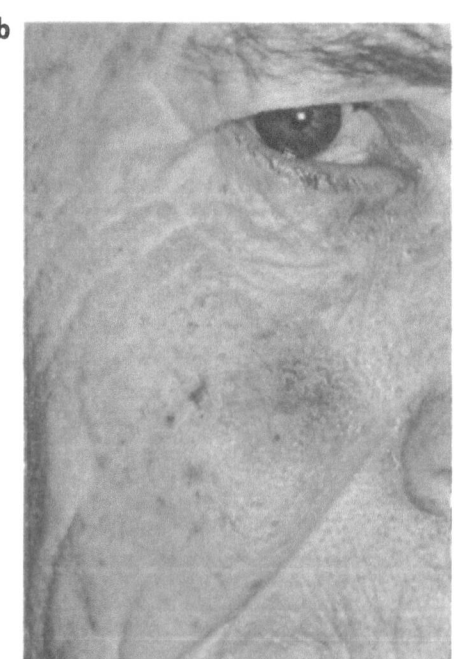

Figure 37. a. Lentigo maligna. **b.** After grenz-ray treatment (individual fractions of 2,000 R daily, total dose 10,000 R; 14.5 kV; $D_{1/2}$, 1.0 mm).

EYE REGION AND EYELIDS

Skin cancers in the eye region are well suited for radiation therapy. Care should be taken to protect the eye during irradiation in order to avoid the most common sequelae, cataract and glaucoma. Functional damage, such as ectropion, also should be prevented.

Lead shielding (see p. 74). After administration of a local anesthetic solution into the conjunctival sac, a lubricated cup-shaped lead shield is inserted under the eyelid (Figs. 29–31; see also Knierer and Schirren 1953; Gladstein 1974). The shield should be disinfected carefully after each use. Prophylaxis of conjunctivitis or keratitis by applying an antibiotic ophthalmic ointment is advisable. The eyelids are a common site of skin cancer. Basal cell cancers are frequently seen in this location (about 60% of all lid tumors are basal cell cancers). They have a predilection for the lower lid and medial canthus. Squamous cell cancers may occur on the upper lid.

Indication. Tumors in this location are a good indication for radiotherapy.

Radiation quality. The radiation quality should correspond to the depth of the tumor. In the area of the medial canthus, slightly more penetrating radiation qualities (HVL, 0.4–0.8 mm Al; $D_{1/2}$, 7–13 mm) are preferred because these carcinomas have a tendency to invade deeply and early. Whenever possible, the area of the lacrimal duct should be shielded to avoid ductal occlusion. However, adequate field size is essential to prevent recurrences. Domonkos (1965) described the results of contact radiation.

Dosage. Single doses of 500 R are suggested up to a total of 5,000 or 6,000 R. At or near the medial canthus, harder radiation qualities and a longer TSD should be used, preferably without increasing the total dose.

Therapeutic results. Permanent cure rates are high (85–95%) (Figs. 32 a and b) and the cosmetic results are very gratifying. Treatment of extensive tumors of the eyelid involves the risk of ectropion or entropion; this rare event can be corrected easily by surgical measures. Obliteration of the lacrimal duct at the medial canthus is often caused by involvement of the duct itself and is difficult to avoid, both with radiation therapy and with surgical measures.

LIPS

Carcinomas of the lip are seen quite frequently in dermatologic practice. Squamous cell cancers prefer the lower lip, showing exophytic or endophytic growth. Depending on the location of the tumor on the medial or lateral aspect of the lower lip, lymph node involvement may be submental or submandibular.

Basal cell cancers have a predilection for the upper lip; they may extend into the vermilion border.

Indication. Radiotherapy offers superior results in the treatment of these tumors (see Fig. 35a and b). The relative merits of surgery and irradiation should be considered in each case. We prefer surgical excision of very small and very large carcinomas of the lip. In addition to size and location of the tumor, the degree of differentiation is an important factor in selecting the proper treatment, as is the age of the patient (see p. 78).

Technique. A sufficiently large field of irradiation is essential. Gums and teeth should be protected with a lead shield (0.5–1 mm thick) covered with a rubber cot. If the tumor is surrounded by precancerous lesions (actinic cheilitis, leukoplakia), these are best included in the treatment area.

Radiation quality. Depending on depth and size of the tumor, soft x rays with a $D_{1/2}$ ranging from 8 to 18 mm may be used (HVL, 0.4–1.4 mm Al; TSD, 15–30 cm).

Dosage. Depending on the rate of tumor involution, total doses may vary from 5,000 to 8,000 R. Single doses of about 500 R are recommended for tumors measuring up to 4 cm in diameter; for larger tumors, doses of 350–400 R are in order. Periodic intermissions of 8–10 days are useful, especially during treatment of large solitary exophytic tumors.

The erosive reaction of the vermilion border is more severe and occurs more rapidly than in other skin areas. The oral mucous membrane often develops an early and painful erosive reaction requiring symptomatic treatment with corticosteroid or anesthetic preparations. The total dosage is governed by the rate of tumor involution as assessed by palpation. Extensive tumors requiring a large field of irradiation should be treated with smaller total dosages.

Therapeutic results. Five-year survival rates are similar for surgery and for radiotherapy (73 and 72%) (Storck et al. 1972). Absence of metastases at the start of treatment is an essential requirement for successful radiotherapy. Histologic examination may be indicated because an enlarged lymph node is not necessarily a metastasis.

Regional lymph node metastasis. If regional metastatic nodes are present, treatment may be surgical (neck dissection), radiotherapeutic (electron beam), or combined (neck dissection preceded or followed by radiotherapy). This type of radiation treatment should be administered by a radiotherapist.

TRUNK

The skin of the trunk has a greater tendency to develop radiation sequelae than the face. When other forms of therapy are unavailable, it is advisable to reduce radiation dosage in order to avoid unsightly chronic radiodermatitis of the treated area (see Fig. 26 a and b on p. 57).

Indication. If a tumor of the trunk is amenable to surgical measures, these should be preferred over radiation therapy. Cosmetic results are usually superior with surgery, unless there is a tendency to keloid formation.

Radiation quality. Selection of radiation follows the general rules (HVL, 0.2–0.4 mm Al; TSD, 30 cm; $D_{1/2}$, 4–8 mm).

Dosage. Single doses of 200–300 R produce better long-term cosmetic results than do larger individual doses. Because a reduction in single dosage requires an increase in total dosage, there are limits as to the minimal individual dose levels one can use. In the area of the spinous processes of the vertebral column, x-ray therapy should be applied with special caution, for aggravation of radiodermatitis by secondary factors with subsequent radiation ulcer or painful scarring is especially common in this region.

EXTREMITIES

In the presence of impaired circulation, the distal extremities tolerate radiation even less than the trunk. In areas such as fingers, toes, and dorsa of feet and hands, the close proximity of bone tissue is another factor limiting the usefulness of x-ray therapy.

Radiation quality. The radiation selected should be of low penetration (e.g., HVL, 0.2 mm Al; TSD, 30 cm; $D_{1/2}$, 4 mm).

Dosage. Single and total dosage should be reduced. A total dose of 8,000 R delivered to the dorsum of the hand may cause severe radiation damage, whereas on the cheek it would be tolerated without adverse effects. Hence, the total dose administered to those sensitive areas should not be higher than 4,000–4,500 R (single fractions, 300–400 R).

Therapeutic Results. Radiation sequelae in these areas are common, especially if the field is larger than 1.5 cm in diameter. Surgical measures are generally preferred.

ANOGENITAL REGION

Radiation therapy in this area should always be preceded by proctoscopy in order to assess the extent of the lesion. The scrotum should be shielded with a lead bag instead of a lead shield. Surgical procedures often yield better results than radiotherapy in these areas. When x-ray therapy is necessary in special cases, the usual principles of tumor radiotherapy apply.

PENIS

Carcinoma of the penis has a predilection for the dorsal aspect of the glans penis, the sulcus coronarius, and the prepuce. The prognosis is poor. Referral to a urologist or radiotherapist is advisable.

VULVA

Squamous cell carcinoma of this region, sometimes secondary to lichen sclerosus et atrophicus, occurs predominantly in older women. Referral to a gynecologist or radiotherapist is advisable. Recently, remarkable results have been obtained with electron beam therapy.

4.3 RADIOTHERAPY OF MALIGNANT MELANOMA

There is considerable controversy regarding the relative merits of surgical, radiotherapeutic, or combined measures in the treatment of malignant melanoma. Statistical evaluation of the therapeutic results obtained with each method is difficult because malignant melanoma may be fatal even after a 5–10 year remission. The prognosis depends on various pathogenetic factors (melanoma arising from a pigmented nevus, unaltered skin, or lentigo maligna), location of the primary tumor, and evidence of metastasis.

In recent years, surgery has been widely accepted as the treatment of choice. We concur in this opinion. Because of the relatively high radioresistance of malignant melanoma, radiotherapy alone has been gradually abandoned (total doses of 12,000–20,000 R are required) (Fig. 25 on p. 56). The combined surgical and radiotherapeutic method calls for a single dose of about 6,000 R to the primary tumor, immediately followed by excision of the entire irradiated area. Prophylactic lymph node excision may be performed at the same time (Hornstein 1972).

Electron beam therapy appears to have produced some favorable results but the data are too incomplete to permit valid conclusions.

4.4 RADIOTHERAPY OF MALIGNANT MESODERMAL NEOPLASMS (SARCOMAS)

Malignant mesodermal neoplasms are considerably less common than malignant epithelial tumors of the skin. Radiotherapeutic results are difficult to evaluate because of the relatively small number of cases reported in the literature and different classifications used by various authors.

FIBROSARCOMA

Surgical methods are preferred over radiotherapy.

DERMATOFIBROSARCOMA PROTUBERANS

See p. 110.

KAPOSI'S SARCOMA (Multiple Idiopathic Hemorrhagic Sarcoma)

See p. 107.

HEMANGIOSARCOMA (Angioplastic Reticulosarcoma)

This very rare disease is virtually resistant to therapy. Therapeutic trials with soft x rays and electron beam (betatron, 2,000–4,500 R) have failed to produce significant results.

MALIGNANT HEMANGIOENDOTHELIOMA

Radiotherapy may be expected to produce more favorable results when the tumors originate in organs other than the skin.

MALIGNANT HEMANGIOPERICYTOMA

Surgical measures are preferred. Palliative treatment with doses of about 3,000 R and tumor doses of 7,000–8,000 R have been recommended.

LYMPHANGIOSARCOMA

This rare type of tumor may develop in edematous tissue following mastectomy (Steward–Treves syndrome). A therapeutic trial by a radiotherapist may be indicated.

LEIOMYOSARCOMA

Radiotherapy may be used as an adjunct to surgery. Electron beam (betatron) therapy would be the first choice among the modalities available.

MYXOSARCOMA

This tumor is rare and therapy resistant. Surgical removal is the treatment of choice. A trial with electron beam (betatron) may be justified.

4.5 RADIOTHERAPY OF CUTANEOUS LYMPHOMAS, RETICULOSES, AND LEUKEMIAS

BENIGN LYMPHOCYTOMA CUTIS (Lymphadenosis Cutis Benigna)

This disease is characterized by benign lymphoreticular hyperplasia of the skin and has a tendency to involute spontaneously. It is highly sensitive to ionizing radiation.

Radiation qualities. Radiation having a $D_{1/2}$ of 3–8 mm (HVL, 0.2–0.4 mm Al; TSD, 15–30 cm) is recommended. Grenz-ray therapy has also been found helpful.

Dosage. Single doses of 100 R, up to a total of 500 R, or three or four single doses of 300 R at 3–4 week intervals, up to a total of 900–1,200 R, have been advocated. In the early stage of the disease, lesions involute rapidly following treatment with small fractions of x rays.

Therapeutic results. Lymphocytoma cutis is a good indication for cutaneous radiotherapy and responds well to treatment.

LYMPHOCYTIC INFILTRATION OF THE SKIN (Jessner and Kanof)

Response to radiation therapy is not unequivocal.

RETICULUM CELL LYMPHOMAS

Cutaneous manifestations of reticuloses and reticulum cell sarcoma usually respond to radiation therapy, particularly when they arise primarily in the skin. There is a strong tendency to recurrence. Radiotherapy should not be instituted without previous biopsy.

Teleroentgentherapy may be used for generalized, flat infiltrating lesions (for technical details, see p. 137). Single doses of 100 R may be given at daily intervals, to a total of 500–1,500 R.

Solitary, deeply infiltrating nodular tumors may be treated with electron beam therapy (betatron).

Indication. This group of disorders responds readily to x rays.

Radiation quality. Small, flat tumors should be treated with soft radiation. The $D_{1/2}$ should equal the tumor depth (HVL, 0.2–1.4 mm Al; TSD, 30 cm.; $D_{1/2}$, 4–18 mm).

Dosage. Single doses of 150–200 R are given four to five times at 2–8 day intervals, up to a total of 800–1,000 R. In cases of reticulum cell sarcoma, higher doses are required (total dose 3,000–5,000 R; interval, 1–2 days).

Therapeutic results. Radiation therapy is the treatment of choice for reticulum cell lymphomas originating in the skin. The prognosis is, nevertheless, unfavorable. Localized forms of malignant cutaneous reticuloses have a better survival rate.

LYMPHOSARCOMA

Either x irradiation or electron beam therapy may be used.

Radiation quality. Soft x rays with a $D_{1/2}$ of 4–18 mm may be administered, depending on the depth of the tumor (HVL, 0.2–1.4 mm Al; TSD, 30 cm).

Dosage. Single doses of 200–350 R are indicated, up to a total of 3,000–4,000 R. The rate of tumor involution may vary considerably from patient to patient.

Therapeutic results. The long-term prognosis is poor. Combined chemotherapy and radiation therapy is frequently required. Consultation with a radiotherapist is advised.

HAND–SCHÜLLER–CHRISTIAN DISEASE

There is usually no indication for radiotherapy in this disorder. Occasionally, temporary improvement of cutaneous lesions has been obtained with soft x rays (HVL, 0.2 mm Al; TSD, 30 cm; $D_{1/2}$, 4 mm) at low dosage (single fractions of 200 R at 2-day intervals, up to a total of 1,000 R).

LETTERER–SIWE DISEASE

This disorder usually is not treated with radiation. Storck (1972) has reported one case where the cutaneous manifestations were treated successfully with soft x rays (29 kV; filter, 0.5 mm Al; HVL, 0.3 mm Al; dose, 7×100 R).

MASTOCYTOSIS (Urticaria Pigmentosa)

Neither solitary mastocytoma nor diffuse mastocytosis are indications for radiation therapy.

MYCOSIS FUNGOIDES

The clinical course of this disease may be divided into three stages: (1) premycotic stage, (2) plaque stage, and (3) tumor stage.

Indication. Next to systemic corticosteroids and cytotoxic drugs, radiation therapy is often the treatment of choice in the management of mycosis fungoides (see Epstein et al. 1972). Although the response of mycosis fungoides lesions to radiation is excellent, recurrences or new lesions cannot be prevented. Because involvement of internal organs usually occurs in the later stages of the disease, dermatologic radiotherapy is often the most important therapeutic modality for patients with this disease over long periods of time. Favorable results have also been obtained in the treatment of extensive lesions with low-energy electron beam therapy at 2.5–5.0 MeV (p. 40) (Fromer et al. 1961) or with topical nitrogen mustard therapy.

In general, mycosis fungoides should not be treated aggressively with ionizing radiation. Because cutaneous lesions frequently become increasingly radioresistant, x rays or electrons are usually used after topical measures have been exhausted (e.g., local corticosteroids, topical nitrogen mustard, UV irradiation).

Therapeutic results. Excellent palliative results may be obtained at all stages of mycosis fungoides (Fig. 36 a and b). Radiotherapy is one of the most effective weapons in the treatment of mycosis fungoides, together with topical nitrogen mustard, UV radiation, topical and systemic corticosteroids, and cytotoxic drugs. Until now the generally accepted rule for radiotherapy of lymphomas was not to exceed the minimal effective dosage. This view has recently been challenged. Early vigorous treatment with topical nitrogen mustard has been advised for long-term palliation. Similarly, total body electron therapy with massive doses (over 3,000 rads) has been advocated in early stages of mycosis fungoides in order to eliminate the disease permanently (Fuks and Bagshaw 1971). It remains to be seen whether long-term follow-up reports are to prove the validity of these new therapeutic concepts.

PREMYCOTIC STAGE

Because of the limited depth of the lesions (which may resemble nondescript dermatitis or psoriasis) grenz rays or slightly filtered soft x rays are usually sufficient. Radiotherapy should be used sparingly at this stage; other forms of therapy should be given preference.

Radiation quality. Grenz rays ($D_{1/2}$, 0.5 mm) or soft x rays having a $D_{1/2}$ of 1.5–2.0 mm are usually adequate.

Dosage. Single doses of 50–200 R may be given three or four times at weekly intervals, up to a total of 200–800 R. When mycosis fungoides presents as generalized erythroderma, teleroentgen therapy is the method of choice. Doses of 50–200 R are delivered daily or at 2-day intervals first to the anterior, then to the posterior surface, up to a total of 500–1,000 R (for technical details, see p. 135).

PLAQUE STAGE

Radiation quality. Slightly more penetrating radiation is required at this stage of the disease. Depending on clinical and histologic findings, soft x rays with a $D_{1/2}$ of 3–10 mm (HVL, 0.1–0.6 mm Al) are recommended.

Dosage. Single doses of 200 R may be given three to five times at 2–8 day intervals, up to a total of 600–1,000 R. Generalized lesions respond very well to teleroentgen therapy (for technical details, see p. 136) or electron beam therapy (p. 40). Single doses of 80–100 R to the anterior and posterior body surfaces are administered daily, up to a total of 1,000–1,500 R (Fig. 38) (see also p. 137). Caution is indicated when cytotoxic drugs are administered concurrently: rapid tumor involution may lead to toxic reactions; periodic blood counts are mandatory.

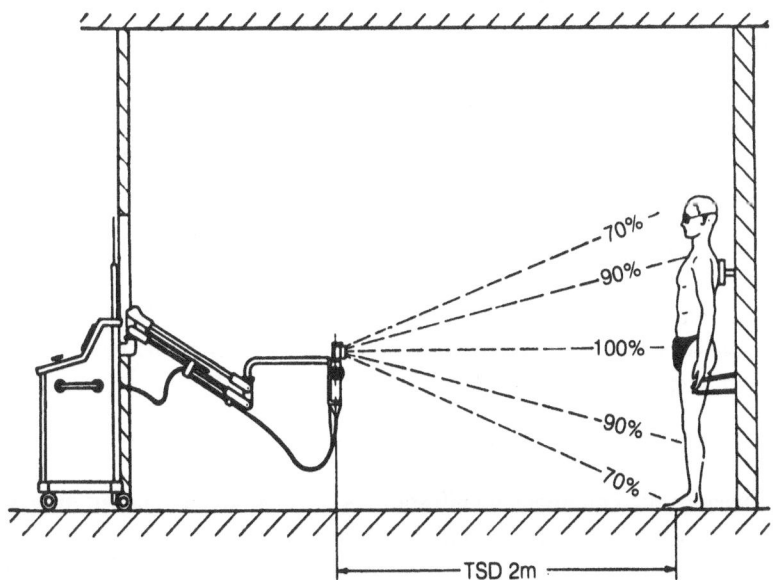

Figure 38. Positioning of patient for teleroentgen therapy. TSD, 2m; relative dose rates in percent. Lead shielding of eyes and gonads (from Schirren 1959).

TUMOR STAGE (Fig. 36 a)

Radiation quality. Soft radiation having a $D_{1/2}$ of 3–18 mm, depending on the depth of the tumor, is indicated (HVL, 0.2–1.4 mm Al; TSD, 30 cm). Adequate field size is essential.

Dosage. Individual tumors are treated with single doses of 150–300 R twice each week until tumor involution is obtained. Total doses generally range from 1,000 to 2,000 R. In generalized cases, electron beam therapy is more suitable than teleroentgen therapy because of its deeper penetration.

In all three stages of mycosis fungoides, it is important to administer minimal therapeutic doses because the cutaneous lesions may become increasingly radioresistant when repeated courses of treatment are administered.

HODGKIN'S DISEASE (Lymphogranulomatosis)

LYMPHOGRANULOMATOSIS CUTIS (Specific Lesions)

The specific maculopapular or nodular lesions vary in their response to radiation therapy.

Radiation quality. Doses of 500–1,000 R are administered in small fractions (150–200 R). Restraint should be used in treating these lesions so that their rate of involution may be assessed correctly. In isolated cases, higher total doses (4,000 R) may be required.

Therapeutic results. The lesions usually respond quite favorably but may vary considerably in their radiosensitivity from case to case. There are no objections to combining chemotherapy with irradiation.

LYMPHOGRANULOMATOSIS CUTIS (Nonspecific Lesions)

Soft x rays effectively control pruritus and eczematoid nonspecific lesions (HVL, 0.2–0.3 mm Al; TSD, 15–30 cm, $D_{1/2}$, 2–5 mm). Three to four doses of 150–200 R are recommended. Encouraging advances have been made recently in the radiotherapy of systemic Hodgkin's disease with megavoltage techniques.

LEUKEMIA CUTIS

Because the cutaneous manifestations of lymphocytic and granulocytic leukemia are similar, they are discussed together.

NONSPECIFIC ECZEMATOUS ERUPTIONS

Eczematous changes respond well to low weekly radiation doses (60–150 R).

Radiation quality. In some cases, grenz rays ($D_{1/2}$, 0.5 mm) may suffice.

Dosage. Single doses of 100–150 R are given three or four times at weekly intervals.

GENERALIZED ERYTHRODERMA

Teleroentgen therapy may be considered (technical details p. 137). Total doses range from 500 to 1,500 R, depending on the clinical response. Electron beam treatments also have palliative value.

SPECIFIC LEUKEMIC TUMORS

These are highly susceptible to x-ray therapy.

Radiation quality. Radiation having a $D_{1/2}$ of 4–18 mm (HVL 0.2–1.4 mm Al; TSD, 30 cm) is usually adequate. Tumors of greater depth may require intermediate therapy (HVL, 2–3 mm Al; TSD, approximately 10 cm) or even orthovoltage therapy ($D_{1/2}$, 5–8 cm; HVL, 0.8–5.0 mm Cu; TSD, 30–50 cm). Referral to a radiotherapist is advisable.

Dosage. After administration of three to four single doses of 150–200 R per day, the rate of tumor involution is evaluated. Treatment is continued for a full tumor dose if the tumors fail to resolve.

4.6 RADIOTHERAPY OF PREMALIGNANT SKIN CONDITIONS

Whereas a number of skin conditions are potentially precancerous, those considered precanceroses in the strict sense of the term include actinic keratoses, leukoplakia, Bowen's disease, Paget's disease, erythroplasia of Queyrat, lentigo maligna, arsenical keratosis, and keratoses associated with xeroderma pigmentosum. Histologically, some of these conditions must be classified as carcinomas *in situ*.

ACTINIC KERATOSIS (Solar Keratosis)

This precancerous condition should be treated primarily by electrodesiccation and curettage, dermabrasion, or 5-fluorouracil. If the biopsy shows carcinomatous degeneration, x-ray therapy may be indicated. The procedure is the same as that described for squamous cell carcinoma (q.v.).

Radiation quality. Soft x rays with thin aluminum filtration and a $D_{1/2}$ of 1–3 mm are preferred. Filtered grenz rays ($D_{1/2}$, 0.8–1.0 mm) have also been used with good cosmetic results (Hollander 1968).

Dosage. Prior to radiation treatment, thick hyperkeratotic scales should be removed with 5% salicylic acid ointment. Individual doses of 800–1,000 R daily, up to a total of 2,000 R, are recommended for fields not exceeding 4 cm in diameter (Storck et al. 1972). For larger fields, 5×400 R are administered at 2- or 3-day intervals. Widespread multiple lesions on forehead and cheeks may be subjected to filtered grenz rays ($D_{1/2}$, 0.8–1.0 mm), $3 \times 1,500$ R (Miescher; cit. in Storck et al. 1972). Topical therapy with 5-fluorouracil is now preferred in most cases.

Therapeutic results. Results are excellent from the clinical as well as the cosmetic point of view. Sun protection is mandatory.

CUTANEOUS HORN (Cornu Cutaneum)

This tumor may develop on the basis of a highly differentiated squamous cell carcinoma, Bowen's disease, or actinic keratosis, or it may be a cutaneous horn in the strict sense of the term. Surgical therapy is preferred. If postoperative radiation therapy is required, the criteria given for squamous cell carcinoma (q.v.) should be observed.

BOWEN'S DISEASE

This precancerous disease of the skin and mucous membranes is highly radiosensitive, as is Bowen's carcinoma (Lukacs 1973; Schoefinius et al. 1974; Hauss et al. 1976). If carcinomatous degeneration is present, radiation therapy should proceed as described under squamous cell carcinoma. Extensive lesions are often suitable for radiotherapy; smaller lesions can be treated adequately with topical 5-fluorouracil or by surgery.

Radiation quality. For selection of radiation quality see Fig. 32. Soft x rays with a $D_{1/2}$ of 2–3 mm are usually adequate (HVL, 0.2 mm Al; TSD, 15–30 cm).

Dosage. Treatment must be continued until an erosive reaction sets in. Fields not exceeding 4 cm in diameter should be irradiated with total doses of 4,000–6,000 R, subdivided into daily doses of 500 R. For larger fields, the individual dose should be reduced to 200–300 R. Radiation protection is of special importance in the genital and anal regions.

Therapeutic results. The treatment is reported to be very effective and the cosmetic results are gratifying.

ERYTHROPLASIA OF QUEYRAT

A number of authors consider erythroplasia of Queyrat and Bowen's disease as identical diseases. Erythroplasia usually occurs on the glans penis or on the prepuce. Because of its low radiosensitivity, this precancerous condition preferably should be treated with surgical measures or topical 5-fluorouracil (Schoefinius et al. 1974).

Radiation quality. Soft x rays with a $D_{1/2}$ of 2–4 mm are recommended (HVL, 0.2–0.3 mm Al; TSD, 15 cm). Gonad protection is important.

Dosage. Erythroplasia usually requires higher total dosages than Bowen's disease. Individual fractions of 300–500 R should be given until an erosive reaction sets in; total dosage may range from 6,000 to 8,000 R.

Therapeutic results. Even though the results are usually satisfactory, other forms of treatment are preferred, particularly for small lesions.

LEUKOPLAKIA

Leukoplakia of the mucous membranes generally has a favorable prognosis. Malignant degeneration is seen in only 10% of the cases. Radiotherapy may be indicated if the biopsy shows malignant degeneration; in this case, the lesion is to be irradiated like a malignant tumor. In general, surgical removal is preferred.

LENTIGO MALIGNA (Hutchinson's Freckle; Melanotic Freckle; Melanosis Circumscripta Praecancerosa of Dubreuilh)

Almost 30% of all malignant melanomas arise from lentigo maligna. This macular lesion occurs predominantly on the exposed areas of the face; it is characterized by slow progression and varied coloration. When nodular lesions are present, transformation to malignant melanoma may have taken place. Melanotic freckle must be differentiated from superficial spreading melanoma.

Indication. Most authors agree that lentigo maligna is eminently suited to superficial radiotherapy, even when the lesion is extensive (Miescher 1955; Arma-Szlachcic et al. 1970; Petratos et al. 1972; Braun-Falco et al. 1975; Hauss et al. 1976). Malignant melanoma or superficial spreading melanoma must be ruled out before treatment is initiated. Kopf et al. (1976) reported metastatic tumors in 3 out of 16 patients treated with the Miescher technique. The use of this procedure has been abandoned in their department.

Radiation quality. Because lentigo maligna is limited to the epidermis, radiation qualities having a $D_{1/2}$ of only 0.5–1 mm are adequate. Treatment of choice is irradiation with filtered grenz rays (14.5 kV; filtered through 1.0 mm Cellon, a plastic material with absorption qualities similar to human skin, or x-ray film; HVL, 0.02 mm Al; TSD, 15 cm; $D_{1/2}$, 1.0 mm).

Dosage. Individual doses of 1,000–2,000 R are given in daily fractions, up to a total of 10,000 R. The erosive reaction is usually characterized by marked exudation.

Therapeutic results. Results are excellent (see Fig. 37 a and b on p. 88) (Lukacs 1973). Occasionally, residual hyperpigmentation caused by melanin deposits in the dermis may require masking with Covermark. These discolorations usually disappear very slowly after 6–12 months.

PAGET'S DISEASE

PAGET'S DISEASE OF THE NIPPLE

Because there is usually an underlying ductal adenocarcinoma, radiotherapy is not advised. Surgical treatment (mastectomy) is always indicated.

EXTRAMAMMARY PAGET'S DISEASE

Radiotherapy is of limited usefulness in this disorder. Because an underlying glandular adnexal carcinoma is frequently associated, surgery is recommended.

Radiation quality. The $D_{1/2}$ should equal the depth of the lesion ($D_{1/2}$, 3–10 mm; HVL, 0.2–0.6 mm Al; TSD, 15–30 cm).

Dosage. Daily fractions of 300–500 R, to a total of 6,000–8,000 R, are recommended.

Therapeutic results. Although successful radiation therapy has been reported, surgical measures should be given preference.

ARSENICAL KERATOSES, RADIOKERATOSES, AND KERATOSES ASSOCIATED WITH XERODERMA PIGMENTOSUM

These precanceroses should not be irradiated because the involved skin has already been damaged by external agents. Surgical excision, electrocoagulation, or similar measures are preferred.

BALANITIS XEROTICA OBLITERANS
(Lichen Sclerosus et Atrophicus Penis)

There is no indication for radiotherapy with this condition.

KRAUROSIS VULVAE (Lichen Sclerosus et Atrophicus Vulvae)

Radiotherapy may be considered as symptomatic antipruritic therapy in elderly patients when other methods have failed (e.g., intralesional cortico-steroid injections).

Radiation quality. Grenz rays are satisfactory.

Dosage. Seventy-five to 100 R may be given at weekly intervals, to a total of 300–500 R. Regular follow-up examinations are required.

Pseudomalignant Lesions

This category includes benign disorders that clinically and histologically resemble squamous cell carcinoma.

FLORID ORAL PAPILLOMATOSIS (Papillomatosis Mucosae Carcinoides)

These verruciform lesions are usually seen on the lips and oral mucosa of older patients, often involving large confluent areas. They are relatively radioresistant and therefore not suitable for radiotherapy. Surgical measures or chemotherapy are preferred.

KERATOACANTHOMA (Molluscum Sebaceum; Self-Healing Epitheliomas [Fergusson-Smith])

These nodular lesions, with characteristic central craters filled with keratin, show a predilection for areas exposed to light. They may occur singly or in groups. Clinical and histologic differentiation from squamous cell carcinomas may be difficult. Instances of malignant degeneration have been described.

Although surgical excision is preferred, an indication for soft x-ray therapy (following biopsy) may exist in some cases where it does not seem advisable to wait for spontaneous involution. The tumor is highly radio-sensitive.

Radiation quality. Depending on size and location of the lesion, soft x rays with a $D_{1/2}$ of 3–12 mm are recommended (HVL, 0.3–1.4 mm Al; TSD, 15 cm).

Dosage. Involution of the tumor may be obtained with as few as three or four doses of 400–500 R each at 1–8 day intervals. If after a total of 2,000–2,500 R no rapid involution is seen, the tumor may be a squamous cell carcinoma. In this case, treatment should be continued according to the criteria given for radiotherapy of carcinomas (q.v.).

Therapeutic results. Fractional x-ray therapy of keratoacanthomas with relatively low total doses often produces satisfactory results. It should be remembered, however, that the rate of spontaneous involution is relatively high.

4.7 RADIOTHERAPY OF BENIGN SKIN TUMORS

Because of advances in other fields of therapy modern indications for radiotherapy of benign skin tumors are limited. Radiation protection measures and safe dose limits are of utmost importance. Radiation sequelae, such as atrophic or pigmentary changes, or telangiectases must be avoided.

Vascular Tumors

HEMANGIOMAS

NEVUS FLAMMEUS (Portwine Stain)

Radiotherapy of nevi flammei with superficial x rays, grenz rays, or thorium X has been largely abandoned because the results have been inconsistent and disappointing.

HEMANGIOMA CAVERNOSUM (Strawberry Mark)

Hemangiomas are benign vascular tumors that may appear at birth or shortly thereafter. Cavernous hemangiomas usually present as sharply circumscribed bluish-red tumors (hemangioma cavernosum cutaneum). They may extend into the subcutis (hemangioma cavernosum cutaneum et subcutaneum) or they may be limited to the subcutis (hemangioma cavernosum subcutaneum). They occur predominantly on the head.

Because most hemangiomas show a tendency to spontaneous involution, x-ray therapy should be limited to exceptional cases. The cutaneous type has a considerably higher rate of spontaneous regression (60–70%) than the subcutaneous type. Under no circumstances should hemangiomas be treated with full tumor doses.

In rare instances of fast-growing and large hemangiomas, cautious x-ray therapy may be administered for the following reasons (see also Witten and Kopf 1959):

> 1. Facial hemangiomas may cause functional or cosmetic impairment. Periorificial hemangiomas are particularly dangerous.

2. Spontaneous regression is sometimes associated with ulceration and scarring, especially in intertriginous areas or in areas subjected to pressure; this may produce unacceptable cosmetic results.
3. Spontaneous regression may take several years. This might cause unsightly permanent pouchlike stretching of the involved area, necessitating surgical repair.

Radiation quality. Soft x rays are preferred (29–50 kV; HVL 0.3–1.4 mm Al; TSD 15–30 cm). The $D_{1/2}$ should closely approximate the depth of the hemangioma, because inhomogeneous irradiation (caused by insufficient $D_{1/2}$) has been reported to stimulate growth.

Dosage. Hemangiomas of up to 4 cm in diameter may be treated with single doses of 150–300 R. Occasionally, one or two treatments with a 6–8 week interval are sufficient. Maximal total dosage is 1,000–1,500 R; smaller total doses are adequate in most cases. If the tumor shows regression after the first treatment, intervals may be increased to 3–4 months. Signs of involution are fading of the intensely red color of the lesion, followed by appearance of grayish-white patches and a reduction in volume. Hemangiomas situated over bone tissue (but not over epiphyses) or lesions measuring more than 4 cm in diameter should be treated with divided doses (e.g., 3 × 100 R at daily intervals) in order to protect the underlying tissue and avoid ulceration.

Important considerations in the treatment of cavernous hemangiomas.

1. Radiotherapy should not be advised as a routine treatment for this condition. Regular follow-up visits and psychologic guidance of the parents are often the only measures required.
2. Where radiation treatment is deemed necessary, it may be instituted at 10–12 weeks of age. In the case of very rapidly growing hemangiomas, age limits should be disregarded.
3. Radiotherapy sessions should be separated by sufficiently long intervals so that involutional changes can be assessed correctly.
4. Deep hemangiomas involving both cutis and subcutis may be compressed with a Cellon disk of 1–2 mm thickness in order to reduce the required $D_{1/2}$. (Cellon is a plastic material with absorption qualities similar to human skin.)
5. In the treatment of rapidly growing hemangiomas, the individual doses should be kept small and given in several fractions (e.g., 300 R subdivided into 3 × 100 R or 6 × 50 R). This will help avoid ulceration.

6. Ulcerated and thrombosed hemangiomas should not be irradiated because they have a pronounced tendency to spontaneous involution.
7. Special consideration should be given to the site of the hemangioma.

Radiotherapy of cavernous hemangiomas in special locations. Extreme caution is indicated in treating hemangiomas near highly radiosensitive structures, such as epiphyses, thyroid, or thymus.

Fontanels. Hemangiomas located near open fontanels should not be irradiated.

Eyelids. In rare instances, hemangiomas of the eyelids may cause blindness. In these cases the eyes should be protected with cup-shaped lead shields to prevent cataracts (see p. 74). Cornea and conjunctiva are anesthetized (see p. 89) before the lead shields are introduced. Fractionation of individual doses is recommended.

Bone growth zones (joints and epiphyses). Irradiation of lesions located in these areas should be avoided whenever possible in order to prevent inhibition of bone growth. If radiotherapy is used, it should be remembered that deep cavernous hemangiomas may cause retardation of bone growth in these locations; therefore, diagnostic x rays should be taken before initiation of radiotherapy. Only superficial radiation should be administered; the $D_{1/2}$ should not exceed 0.6–1.0 mm. Subdivision of dosage (e.g., into 50-R fractions; see above) is recommended.

Mammary glands, thymus, thyroid region, and gonads (testes, ovaries). Hemangiomas in these areas should not be exposed to radiation. Atrophy of the breast, benign thyroid tumors, and thyroid cancers may occur many years later.

Therapeutic results. Gratifying results may be obtained with soft x rays, provided that good judgment has been used both in selecting the treatment and in applying it. Before he or she decides on the appropriate form of treatment, the therapist should consider the strong tendency to spontaneous involution of cutaneous cavernous hemangiomas and the final cosmetic result to be expected.

PYOGENIC GRANULOMA

Surgical methods are superior to radiotherapy and should be given preference.

GLOMUS TUMOR (Glomangioma)

This tumor does not respond well to radiotherapy. Some favorable results have been reported, however (5 $\times$ 400 R; $D_{1/2}$, 7 mm; HVL, 0.4 mm Al; TSD, 30 cm).

KAPOSI'S SARCOMA

Favorable results can be obtained when radiotherapy is instituted in the early stages of the illness.

Radiation quality. Soft x rays, with a $D_{1/2}$ equal to the depth of the individual lesions.

Dosage. Single doses of 200–300 R, up to a total dose of 1,000 R; rarely up to 2,000–3,000 R.

Therapeutic results. Thirty-five percent of 94 patients showed complete remissions (Storck et al. 1972). The long-term prognosis is clouded, however, by the well-known tendency of this disease to recurrences, even after intervals of several years.

Tumors of the Lymphatic Vessels

LYMPHANGIOMAS

Lymphangiomas are benign tumors composed of lymphatic vessels; occasionally, they contain vascular elements (hemolymphangioma). They occur considerably less frequently than hemangiomas and reports on radiotherapeutic results are rare.

The superficial circumscribed type (lymphangioma circumscriptum cysticum) consists of discrete, translucent lesions resembling vesicles. Preferred sites are tongue, extremities, and trunk.

The cavernous type (lymphangioma cavernosum subcutaneum) presents deeper and larger lesions, which often involve an entire part of the body. Both forms appear at birth or in early infancy and show no spontaneous involution; occasionally, they may significantly increase in size.

Treatment. Because lymphangiomas have little tendency to grow, their radiosensitivity, as compared to that of hemangiomas, is very low. Some authors consider them radioresistant. The cavernous subcutaneous forms are said to respond somewhat more favorably than the superficial lesions. Improvement following treatment with beta radiation has been reported (Cipollaro and Crossland 1967).

Radiation quality. When surgical removal is not feasible, radiotherapy of cavernous lymphangiomas may be tried, provided the dose can be delivered to the deeper portions of the lesion without damage to the surrounding tissues. In these cases, the same principles apply as in radiotherapy of hemangiomas: Treatment should be initiated in the early stages of the tumor; soft x rays are preferred (HVL, 0.2–1.4 mm Al; TSD, 15–30 cm; $D_{1/2}$, 3–18 mm). The $D_{1/2}$ should equal the estimated depth of the lesion. Electron beam treatment may also be considered.

Dosage. Individual doses are similar to those used in hemangioma (3–4 $\times$ 200–300 R); intervals between treatments are shorter. Late radiation sequelae must be avoided.

If electron beam (betatron) treatment is used, a dosage of 3–4 $\times$ 300 R at daily intervals is recommended (Bode 1970).

Therapeutic results. Although x-ray treatment of circumscribed and cavernous lymphangiomas is not generally advocated, a trial may be worthwhile in some cases. Favorable results have been reported with electron beam treatments of cavernous lymphangiomas. On the whole, the results of radiotherapy in the treatment of lymphangiomas have been unsatisfactory.

Tumors of the Connective Tissue

KELOIDS

There is general agreement that primary or postoperative radiotherapy or intralesional injections of corticosteroids are useful in the treatment of keloids (Domonkos 1971). Since the therapeutic effect of irradiation is the same in spontaneous keloids and in keloids developing in scars, it is not necessary to discuss these two types separately. Both must be differentiated, however, from hypertrophic scars, which resolve spontaneously.

The radiosensitivity of keloids depends largely on their age. New, fast-growing keloids resolve quite rapidly after irradiation. Results are best when treatment is instituted during the first 6 months after appearance of the keloid.

RADIOTHERAPY OF LARGE AND SMALL KELOIDS

Duration of the condition is an important factor in selecting the treatment of small keloids. Keloids of more than 6 months duration usually respond less readily to x rays. Growths that are more than 2 years old are largely resistant to radiotherapy.

Treatment of large keloids with radiotherapy alone is basically the same as that of small keloids; the individual doses, however, are smaller (e.g., 200 R).

Radiation quality. The $D_{1/2}$ should be equal to the depth of the lesion, the field size to its area.

Dosage. Total dosage should be 1,000–1,200 R. In special cases, up to 2,500 R may be given, but possible late sequelae have to be anticipated. In general, individual doses of 300–400 R are given at 4-week intervals. If the growth does not respond appreciably after three (or four) treatments, further radiotherapy holds little promise.

Therapeutic results. In small, early keloids, fractional soft x-ray therapy is often effective. Duration and size of the keloid are prime determinants in the selection of treatment. Eighty percent of small keloids developing after surgery respond well to radiotherapy, whereas large keloids show a favorable response in only 50% of the cases.

POSTOPERATIVE RADIOTHERAPY IN COMBINATION WITH CORTICOSTEROID THERAPY

Large keloids and those that are more than 6 months old are less suited to radiotherapy alone (Schirren 1959 a); for these cases, some authors recommend surgical excision followed by irradiation. Radiotherapy should be used only if there is evidence of new keloid formation after the wound has healed. It is doubtful whether prophylactic x irradiation of a surgical scar immediately after removal of the sutures can prevent keloid development (Cipollaro and Crossland 1967; Grover 1965).

When intralesional injections alone are unsuccessful, the method of choice may be intralesional injection of corticosteroids followed by radiotherapy.

Radiation quality. The surrounding normal tissue must be shielded with lead foil to the very edge of the lesion. With regard to radiation quality, the criteria are the same as with radiotherapy alone ($D_{1/2}$ equals depth of keloid). Radiation qualities ranging from 29 to 50 kV are usually satisfactory (0.4–1.0 mm Al added filter; HVL, 0.3–0.9 mm Al; $D_{1/2}$, 3–12 mm).

Dosage. The dosage for postoperative radiotherapy of small keloids is the same as with primary irradiation. We recommend three to four doses of 300–400 R at 4-week intervals, up to a total dose of 1,000–1,200 R (only in exceptional cases up to 2,000 R).

Some authors have treated keloids with daily to weekly fractional doses, starting 7–14 days after excision. Single doses of 200 R were given, up to a total of 1,800–2,500 R. These doses may lead to undesirable sequelae, particularly atrophy and teleangiectases.

When radiation treatment is started immediately after the surgical wound has healed, four daily doses of 300 R have been recommended (50 kV; HVL, 0.8 mm Al; TSD, 15–30 cm; $D_{1/2}$, 12–13 mm). Treatment with harder radiation (140 kV; HVL, 2.0 mm Al; TSD, 25 cm) is not advisable.

Therapeutic results. Surgical excision of keloids alone often results in extensive recurrences. In the past, radiotherapy was the only method that prevented such recurrences and, at the same time, produced excellent cosmetic results. More recently, very satisfactory results have been obtained with intralesional injections of corticosteroids. The prevailing view at the present time is that x-ray treatment should be given only after an unsuccessful trial of intralesional steroids.

DERMATOFIBROSARCOMA PROTUBERANS

This locally aggressive tumor has a strong tendency to recurrence but rarely metastasizes. Surgical treatment is preferred to radiotherapy.

Benign Epithelial Tumors

SEBORRHEIC KERATOSES (Verrucae Seniles)

Radiotherapy of seborrheic warts is not recommended. The dosage required to induce involution of these benign tumors is relatively high (>1,000 R). Other forms of treatment yield better results.

TRICHOEPITHELIOMA (Epithelioma Adenoides Cysticum)

Minute to pea-sized yellowish nodules in symmetrical distribution occur predominantly in the nasolabial folds. There is usually a family history; onset is in childhood. Radiosensitivity is significantly lower than that of basal cell epitheliomas. Radiotherapy is rarely indicated.

Radiation quality. The normally necessary $D_{1/2}$ of 5–10 mm (HVL, 0.3–0.6 mm Al; TSD, 30 cm) can be reduced if treatment is preceded by surgical planing of raised lesions.

Dosage. Daily doses of 300–400 R, to a total dose of 3,000–5,000 R are required.

Therapeutic results. With the high dosage required, late sequelae (abnormalities of pigmentation, atrophy, teleangiectases) must be expected. This form of therapy is useful only when surgery is contraindicated.

110

PILOMATRICOMA (Calcifying Epithelioma of Malherbe)

There is no indication for radiotherapy with this condition.

CYLINDROMA (Spiegler Tumor)

These are multiple nodular tumors of the scalp, occasionally associated with trichoepitheliomas.

Most authors oppose radiotherapy because of the relatively high radioresistance of these lesions (about 30% higher than that of trichoepitheliomas). Although surgical excision is preferred, radiotherapy may be indicated in selected cases.

Radiation quality. The $D_{1/2}$ should equal the depth of the tumor.

Dosage. Single doses of 300–500 R, totaling up to 4,000–8,000 R may be administered. In the scalp area, potential effects on the brain should be taken into consideration.

Therapeutic results. The treatment is moderately effective, but surgical removal is preferred.

5

Radiotherapy
of benign dermatoses

5.1 GENERAL CONSIDERATIONS

The range of indications for radiotherapy of benign dermatoses has become more and more limited in recent years (Goldschmidt 1959). This is primarily because of the development of other effective local and systemic therapeutic agents, particularly antibiotics and corticosteroids. Fear of radiation side effects became an important contributing factor when the incidence of serious radiation sequelae increased dramatically following the indiscriminate use of ionizing radiation for benign disorders during the first decades of this century (Epstein 1965; Grover 1965).

Dermatologic radiotherapy of benign skin conditions is justified only when there is absolutely no possibility of somatic or genetic damage. Where such a risk exists, radiotherapy is contraindicated. In addition, x rays should be used in most instances only when nonradiative treatment is unavailable or unsuccessful. Establishing an indication for radiation treatment of dermatoses is a complex and responsible task; it requires dermatologic expertise as well as familiarity with radiophysical concepts. The most important aspects are summarized in Table 13.

- Efficient use of radiation is an important prerequisite in the treatment of dermatoses; this criterion is met by selecting a radiation quality having a $D_{1/2}$ equal to the estimated depth of the lesion.
- Only the involved area should be exposed to radiation.
- The minimum effective dose should not be exceeded.
- The maximum permissible dose per area and lifetime should

113

TABLE 13

RADIOTHERAPY OF BENIGN DERMATOSES

Criteria for selecting radiotherapy
1. Establish proper diagnosis before radiotherapy.
2. Administer x rays only when other types of therapy are unsuccessful or unlikely to give relief.
3. Do not use ionizing radiation in children.

Technical aspects of radiotherapy
1. Select technique appropriate for site and depth of lesion.
2. Use minimum effective dosage.
3. Do not exceed maximum permissible dose per area and lifetime.
4. Observe special rules for specific body areas (gonads, face, scalp, etc.).

be observed (800–1,000 R per area, administered in small 60–100 R fractions at long intervals in the course of a lifetime).

- Location of the lesion is an essential factor in determining the potential risk to gonads, eyes, thyroid and hemopoietic system.
- Concomitant topical therapy of the irradiated lesions with potential irritants (e.g., tar or sulfur products) should be avoided.

There are numerous theories concerning the mode of action of x rays in the treatment of benign dermatoses. In most cases, their application is based strictly on empirical knowledge. Following are some of the theories that have been advanced:

1. Enzymatic theory. X rays induce enzymatic effects by releasing antiinflammatory substances from destroyed leukocytes; this stimulates phagocytotic activity, thus accelerating the healing process.
2. Radiation inhibits allergic mechanisms, acting on lymphocytes and possibly on antibody receptors.
3. Theory of neuroregulation. Ionizing radiation acts on the terminal reticulum of the autonomous nervous system and on the sympathetic ganglia, triggering a nonspecific response that restores normal conditions.
4. Radiation-induced destruction of leukocytes converts inflammatory acidosis of the tissue to alkalosis; electrolyte balance is restored and osmotic conditions are normalized; degradation products of the inflammatory process are me-

tabolized more rapidly, and pain produced by acidosis is alleviated.

5. Epidermal and dermal hypertrophy and hyperplasia are reduced by inhibition of mitosis.

6. Enzyme systems and membranes are normalized (repair effect).

These hypotheses indicate that at the present there is no universally accepted theory regarding the mechanism of action of x rays in the treatment of dermatoses (Grover 1965).

5.2 SPECIFIC INDICATIONS

Viral Infections

WARTS—VERRUCAE VULGARES,
VERRUCAE PLANAE JUVENILES, VERRUCAE PLANTARES

Indication. Therapeutic alternatives to x rays are preferred. The lesions are not very radiosensitive, and therapeutically effective doses may cause radiation sequelae. Because warts are frequently located near epiphyses, radiation treatment is contraindicated in children. Undoubtedly, some favorable results obtained with radiotherapy are caused either by spontaneous healing or by psychologic factors.

Although strict adherence to safety standards can yield favorable therapeutic results without sequelae, routine irradiation of verrucae vulgares, verrucae plantares, and verrucae planae juveniles is not recommended. Rare exceptions include treatment of resistant plantar warts. The $D_{1/2}$ should equal the depth of the lesion (HVL, 0.3 mm Al; TSD, 30 cm; $D_{1/2}$, 4 mm).

Dosage. Single doses of 200–300 R at 2–3 week intervals are recommended (Baer and Witten 1956). In general, the total dosage should not exceed 800–1,000 R in order to avoid radiation sequelae. Pipkin and Lehmann (1949) reported good results with a single-dose technique, administering over 1,000–1,500 R to well-shielded plantar warts up to 2 cm in diameter (Domonkos 1971).

In children with verrucae planae juveniles, pseudo-irradiation might be used. In a remarkably high percentage of the cases, simply "going through the motions" of radiotherapy without actually administering radiation can cause the warts to disappear.

CONDYLOMATA ACUMINATA

There is no indication for radiotherapy with this condition.

HERPES SIMPLEX

Recent reports indicate that radiotherapy may be effective in the acute stage of locally recurrent herpes simplex (Knight 1972). It is conceivable that the favorable results are caused by radiation-induced immunologic mechanisms.

Radiation quality. Soft x rays having a $D_{1/2}$ of 3–4 mm (HVL, 0.2 mm Al; TSD, 15–30 cm) or grenz rays ($D_{1/2}$, 0.5 mm, HVL, 0.03 mm Al) may be used.

Dosage. Single doses of 100–150 R administered on two or three consecutive days, or grenz rays at a dosage of 4×200 R at daily intervals, are recommended. Treatment should coincide with the beginning of the vesicular eruption.

Therapeutic results. Radiotherapy allegedly reduces the frequency and intensity of recurrences. Some authors have reported significant improvement in 80% of their cases following grenz-ray therapy.

HERPES ZOSTER

There is no indication for radiation therapy with this condition.

Bacterial Infections

INDICATION

Radiotherapy of infectious dermatoses is often referred to as antiinflammatory radiotherapy. Indications for antiinflammatory radiotherapy are not limited to the skin but include inflammatory diseases of other organ systems. Relatively small doses are used in this type of irradiation. The number of infectious dermatoses treated with radiotherapy has decreased considerably since the advent of antibiotics.

The guidelines for antiinflammatory radiotherapy of dermatoses are similar to those given on p. 113. Irradiation of inflammatory skin diseases is now used only in rare instances as supportive treatment in combination with systemic drugs (antibiotics, etc.). It is especially valuable in cases where a sufficiently high tissue level of antibiotics is difficult to establish.

The field size should correspond to the extent of the inflammatory changes. The surrounding area must be shielded with a lead shield.

The gonads should be protected with lead rubber shields (details see

p. 63). It should be remembered that harder radiation qualities may cause indirect damage to the gonads. For this reason, more penetrating radiation should be avoided.

As for timing of the treatment, radiotherapy should be started as early as possible in order to produce satisfactory results.

Radiation quality. Soft or superficial x-ray therapy is adequate for all bacterial skin diseases. Again, radiation is used efficiently only if its $D_{1/2}$ corresponds to the depth of the lesion.

Dosage. In antiinflammatory therapy, single doses usually vary between 50 and 150 R. A more acute inflammatory process and a large field of irradiation call for lower single doses than do more chronic processes and smaller fields. Currently, two to four doses of 50–100 R at daily or several days' intervals are favored. In chronic cases, single doses of 100–200 R may be administered, up to a total of 1,000 R.

CUTANEOUS TUBERCULOSIS

Radiotherapy is no longer important in the treatment of the various types of cutaneous tuberculosis. In exceptional cases, it may be used as an adjunct in the treatment of tuberculosis cutis verrucosa (HVL, 0.2–0.4 mm Al; TSD, 30 cm; $D_{1/2}$, 4–7.5 mm).

Dosage. Single doses of 500 R were given at intervals of several days up to a total of 1,500–2,000 R.

LEPROSY

Indications for radiotherapy with this condition are very limited. Treatment is given as in tuberculosis.

RHINOSCLEROMA

Radiation treatment has been recommended occasionally as an adjunct to systemic antibiotics. [Radiation quality: 120 kV; HVL, 3 mm Al; dosage, 400 R three to five times at 4-week intervals, to a total of 1,200–2,000 R (Cipollaro and Crossland 1967)]. Contact therapy with tumor doses has also been recommended.

PYODERMAS

TEMPORARY X-RAY EPILATION

In the preantibiotic era, temporary roentgen epilation was used primarily in fungus infections of the scalp, certain types of folliculitis barbae, chronic folliculitis of the neck (folliculitis sclerotisans nuchae, acne keloidalis), and hidradenitis suppurativa of the axillae. There is no indication for radiotherapy with folliculitis barbae. In the past, temporary x-ray epilation was the accepted method of treating folliculitis decalvans. This is no longer advocated.

Radiation quality. Soft or superficial x rays having a $D_{1/2}$ of 7.5–13 mm (HVL, 0.4–1 mm Al; TSD, 30 cm) are suitable for epilation.

Dosage. For total epilation of the scalp, a single dose of 350–400 R is administered to each of four or five overlapping areas (Kienboeck–Adamson technique). Hairs in the irradiated area are shed approximately 3 weeks after treatment, and regrowth starts 8–10 weeks following irradiation.

Possible adverse effects of improper temporary epilation techniques are pigment changes of the scalp hair, incomplete regrowth of hair, permanent alopecia, radiodermatitis, radiation ulcer, growth retardation of the cranium, as well as eye, thyroid, and brain damage (Modan et al. 1974). These risks can be avoided by taking the proper precautions.

For details concerning the technical procedure, Wagner (1959) or Cipollaro and Crossland (1967) should be consulted.

ACNE KELOIDALIS (Folliculitis Sclerotisans Nuchae)

In the past, roentgen epilation ($D_{1/2}$, 7–11 mm; HVL, 0.4–0.8 mm Al; TSD, 15–30 cm) was widely used for this disease. Today, this method has a place only in cases refractory to other forms of therapy.

FURUNCLES

Indication. Radiotherapy may rarely be indicated as an adjunct to antibiotics in the treatment of furuncles in special locations, particularly in the facial area. Furuncles in other locations usually do not require supportive x-ray therapy.

Radiation quality. A radiation quality suited to the depth of the lesions should be selected; in general, a $D_{1/2}$ of 7–13 mm (HVL, 0.4–0.8 mm Al; TSD, 15–30 cm) is adequate.

Dosage. Daily single doses of 50 (to 80) R are given three or four times.

Therapeutic results. In special cases, radiotherapy is considered a valuable supportive measure by many authors.

118

CARBUNCLES

Radiation therapy is indicated only in exceptional cases as an adjunct to other forms of therapy, particularly in the early stages of the disease. (For radiation quality and dosage, see "Furuncles.")

HIDRADENITIS SUPPURATIVA (Apocrine Abscess)

The preferred site of this staphylococcal infection of the apocrine glands is the axillary region.

Indication. Radiotherapy still has a limited place in the treatment of this disease. Many modern authors consider special cases of hidradenitis suppurativa a valid indication for radiation treatment, particularly when used in combination with systemic antibiotics.

ACUTE HIDRADENITIS

In new acute cases, institution of radiation therapy within 24–48 hours after onset of the disease produces the best results.

Radiation quality. Depending on the depth of the apocrine abscesses, radiation having a $D_{1/2}$ of 10–18 mm (HVL, 0.8–1.4 mm Al; TSD, 15–30 cm) may be selected.

Dosage. Two to three doses of 60–80 R given at 1–2 day intervals are usually recommended.

CHRONIC RECURRENT HIDRADENITIS

Radiation quality. See "Acute Hidradenitis."

Dosage. Small doses (50–100 R) are given in daily fractions until a total surface dose of 400 R (epilation dose) has been reached. Some authors advise a single epilation dose of 400–500 R.

Therapeutic results. Favorable results are obtained in combination with antibiotics. Radiotherapy alone is no longer used in this disease.

ERYSIPELAS

Antiinflammatory radiotherapy used to be a life-saving measure in this now rare disease. It is no longer indicated.

CHRONIC PARONYCHIA

Indication. X-ray therapy has been recommended as an adjunct in the management of chronic paronychia caused by bacterial or *Candida* infection.

Radiation quality. Radiation having a $D_{1/2}$ of 4–8 mm (HVL, 0.2–0.4 mm Al; TSD, 30 cm) is recommended.

Dosage. Single doses of 50–200 R may be given at 3–7 day intervals, up to a maximum of 800 R.

Therapeutic results. Favorable results have been reported, depending on various factors.

Protozoal Infections

CUTANEOUS LEISHMANIASIS

Indication. Only exceptional therapy-resistant cases should be selected for radiation therapy. In the presence of deep infiltrates, x rays may be used as supportive therapy in combination with the usual chemotherapeutic and topical measures.

Radiation quality. Soft x rays with a $D_{1/2}$ of 7.5–13 mm, depending on the depth of the lesions, are indicated (HVL, 0.4–0.8 mm Al; TSD, 30 cm).

Dosage. Three doses of 50–150 R are suggested at 10-day intervals.

Therapeutic results. This method used as supportive therapy reportedly is effective in reducing potential scar formation.

Fungal Infections

TINEAS

Since the advent of effective systemic and local antifungal agents, radiation therapy is no longer required in the treatment of these disorders.

DEEP MYCOSES

ACTINOMYCOSIS

Actinomycosis is caused by funguslike higher bacteria. It is discussed here because it resembles mycoses clinically.

Indication. Radiotherapy should be considered only in combination with systemic therapy.

Radiation quality. Deep colliquative lesions usually require radiation having a $D_{1/2}$ of 1–2 cm. Lesions of still greater depth may require a $D_{1/2}$ of 3 cm.

Dosage. Daily single doses of 200 R, up to a total of 2,000 R, have been recommended in the past. Today, most radiotherapists prefer an antiinflammatory type of treatment with smaller doses (50–100 R, three to four times at daily intervals; treatment may be repeated if necessary).

Therapeutic results. The results are difficult to evaluate with concomitant antibiotic treatment.

BLASTOMYCOSIS AND SPOROTRICHOSIS

Radiation therapy of these disorders has been largely abandoned. In rare instances, favorable results have been obtained in combination with other measures. The techniques are the same as in actinomycosis.

Dermatitis and Eczema

GENERAL INDICATIONS

Various forms of eczematous dermatitis still provide the most common indication for the use of x rays in benign skin diseases. When contemplating radiotherapy, one should consider the etiology, stage, and localization of the disease, as well as the age of the patient, the risk of genetic damage, and previous dermatologic therapy (Goldschmidt 1959). Radiotherapy is most efficacious in lichen simplex chronicus (neurodermatitis circumscripta), psoriasiform dermatitis, and eczematous lesions in special locations. Since the introduction of topical and systemic steroids the use of x rays has decreased dramatically. Radiotherapy is now considered a valuable tool, often as supportive therapy, in the treatment of a limited number of cases of eczema not sufficiently responsive to other types of therapy.

Roentgen rays have been used in the therapy of eczematous dermatoses practically since their discovery. It was soon found that relatively small doses induce involution of the lesions and also control itching. Obviously, x rays are not curative in all cases and recurrences are not uncommon. Unfortunately, it was recognized only decades later that repeated treatments beyond a certain total dose might cause chronic radiation sequelae. The maximum cumulative total dose of 1,000 R (in fractional doses of 60–100 R) must not be exceeded (Sulzberger et al., 1952) (see also p. 65). The recommended cumulative dose for ultrasoft x rays (grenz rays) is in the range of 5,000 R (Pillsbury et al., 1956).

TECHNICAL PROCEDURE

Not every special technique used in the radiation treatment of eczemas can be discussed here. The dose is dependent on the clinical characteristics and the stage of the disease. Eczemas in the acute stage should not be irradiated. Prime indications for radiotherapy are chronic eczematous conditions with pronounced acanthosis, hyperkeratosis, and inflammatory cell proliferation.

Radiation quality. Soft radiation having a $D_{1/2}$ suited to the depth of infiltration (3–4 mm) is recommended (HVL, usually 0.2–0.3 mm Al; TSD, 15–30 cm). Grenz rays ($D_{1/2}$, 0.5 mm; HVL, 0.03 mm Al) may be considered for superficial lesions.

Dosage. A course of three or four individual doses of 60–100 R may be administered weekly. In order to avoid exceeding the safe limits for cumulative dosages, an accurate history should be taken of any previous radiation treatments. In general, not more than two courses of treatment should be given per year, preferably with intervals of more than 3 months. The total dose per area and lifetime should not exceed 1,000 R. Grenz rays are usually given in doses of 150–300 R.

ALLERGIC CONTACT DERMATITIS

Acute and subacute forms of this disorder provide no indication for radiotherapy.

CHRONIC LICHENIFIED ECZEMAS

Stubborn eczematous lesions are excellent indications for radiotherapy when other topical or systemic measures have failed. Residual infiltrates of chronic eczemas respond especially well to x rays.

Radiation quality and dosage. For radiation quality and dosage, see above.

Therapeutic results. Immediate results are usually good. Recurrences can often be prevented with appropriate local supportive measures.

HYPERKERATOTIC TYLOTIC ECZEMA

This eczematous condition has a predilection for the palms and the soles. Opinion varies concerning the value of radiation treatment. We have seen favorable results in a number of cases. Avoid concurrent topical treatment with potentially irritating keratolytic agents or tar preparations.

Radiation quality. Soft x rays with a $D_{1/2}$ of 2–3 mm are favored (HVL, 0.2 mm Al; TSD, 15–30 cm). In the presence of a thick keratotic layer, a $D_{1/2}$ of 4–6 mm may be indicated (HVL, 0.3 mm Al; TSD, 15–30 cm). Grenz rays ($D_{1/2}$, 0.5 mm; HVL, 0.03 mm Al) are less effective, even with higher doses.

Dosage. A course of treatment consists of three or four doses of 75–100 R administered at weekly intervals, to a total of 300–400 R. Not more than two or three courses per area are recommended. If the response is unimpressive there is no point in increasing the dosage. The patient should be questioned specifically about previous radiation treatment.

Therapeutic results. There are negative as well as positive reports. On the whole, radiation therapy seems to be well worth a trial after other topical measures have proved unsuccessful, especially when the condition interferes with daily life.

LICHENIFIED PRIMARY IRRITANT DERMATITIS

Persistent primary irritant dermatitis may result in lichenification. The irritant should be identified and removed before radiotherapy is considered. In our experience, radiation treatment is of limited value in this type of dermatitis.

ONYCHODYSTROPHY SECONDARY TO ECZEMA

Indication. Radiation therapy should be reserved for stubborn, refractory cases.

Radiation quality. For guidelines see p. 122.

Dosage. Single doses of 75–100 R at weekly intervals, up to a total of 225–300 R, are delivered to the nail and the perionychial tissue.

SEBORRHEIC ECZEMA

Radiation treatment of this chronic recurrent dermatosis, which has a predilection for scalp, external auditory canal, retroauricular region, and chest, should be approached with considerable reservations. Only in exceptional cases, particularly in elderly patients where the lesions are few in number and circumscribed, should irradiation be contemplated (see p. 121).

Therapeutic results. Favorable results have been obtained in retroauricular lesions and in psoriasiform and pityriasiform eczematous lesions. Relapses are common.

GENERALIZED SEBORRHEIC ECZEMA

Beneficial results obtained with teleroentgen therapy in rare refractory cases of generalized seborrheic eczema are discussed elsewhere (see p. 138).

Radiation quality. Soft radiation is administered in the form of teleroentgen therapy (50 kV; TSD 2 m; no filtration; $D_{1/2}$, 2 mm).

Dosage.   Single doses of 50 R are given to one aspect of the body surface at 2-day intervals; total doses of 350–500 R have been recommended.

Therapeutic results.   The results are excellent, but relapses are unavoidable.

NUMMULAR ECZEMA

Radiotherapy is of questionable value in this disorder. Therapeutic alternatives should be tried before radiation treatment is considered in exceptionally recalcitrant cases.

Technique.   For radiation quality and dosage, see p. 122.

Therapeutic results.   The frequency of recurrences apparently is not influenced by radiation treatment.

LICHEN SIMPLEX CHRONICUS (Localized Neurodermatitis)

Radiotherapy may be indicated in highly pruritic lesions after corticosteroids or other therapeutic measures have been unsuccessful (see indications for radiotherapy of dermatoses, p. 113, 121).

Radiation quality.   Soft x rays with a $D_{1/2}$ of 2–4 mm (HVL, 0.2 mm Al; TSD, 15–30 cm) may be used. Grenz rays ($D_{1/2}$, 0.5 mm; HVL, 0.03 mm Al) have been successful in some cases but are less suitable for markedly lichenified lesions.

Dosage.   Single doses of 75–100 R are given weekly over a period of 3 or 4 weeks. A second course may be administered 4–6 weeks later. The total dose per area and lifetime must not exceed 1,000 R. The individual doses are doubled when grenz rays are used.

Therapeutic results.   Rapid improvement is often obtained. Pruritus frequently subsides after the first treatment. However, relapses occur in about 50% of the patients. Hence, this modality should be reserved for selected cases.

NEURODERMATITIS; ATOPIC ECZEMA

In view of the intermittent course of the disease and the uncertain therapeutic response, radiotherapy of disseminate neurodermatitis is not advisable. When irradiating rare, highly pruritic, refractory cases, one should remember that these patients tend to change doctors frequently and may deliberately neglect to report previous x-ray therapy. For details concerning radiation treatment of circumscribed lesions, see p. 122.

INFANTILE ECZEMA

Because of the risk of genetic damage, eczematous eruptions in infants and children should not be irradiated. Advances in topical dermatologic therapy have made radiation treatment entirely dispensable.

Papulosquamous Dermatoses

PSORIASIS VULGARIS

Indication. Psoriasis lesions are radiosensitive and respond well to radiotherapy (Harber, 1958). Because of their tendency to recurrence, the following criteria should be observed:

1. Radiotherapy should be considered only as a last resort in exceptionally refractory, inveterate, and distressing cases of psoriasis after other therapeutic possibilities have been exhausted.
2. Only minimum effective doses should be administered (p. 113).
3. Previous x-ray treatments must be evaluated. The maximum cumulative dose per area should never exceed 1,000 R.
4. In children and adolescents, radiotherapy is contraindicated.
5. Acute guttate psoriasis is not suitable for radiation treatment [radiation may even induce an isomorphic response (Koebner effect)].
6. Psoriatic nail changes respond relatively well to radiation treatment.

Radiation quality. Infiltrated lesions may be controlled by soft radiation (HVL, 0.2–0.3 mm Al; TSD, 15–30 cm; $D_{1/2}$, 3–4 mm). However, most superficial lesions respond well to grenz rays with a $D_{1/2}$ of 0.5 mm (HVL, 0.03 mm Al).

Dosage. Individual doses of 75–150 R (soft x rays) are given three or four times at weekly intervals; one or two courses of treatment may be administered per year, preferably with intervals of at least 3 months. When grenz rays are used the corresponding individual doses are higher (200–300 R).

Psoriatic erythroderma often responds well to teleroentgen therapy (50 kV; TSD, 2 m; no filtration); single doses of 50 R are given at 2–3 day intervals to both the frontal and the dorsal body surface, up to a total of 350–600 R (for details see p. 138).

REGIONAL PSORIASIS

Elbows and knees.   Irradiation of the typical predilection sites of psoriasis on elbows and knees is discouraged because of the well-known tendency to recurrence. However, when x rays are used judiciously and the maximum permissible dose per area and lifetime is not exceeded, there is no valid objection to radiation therapy of obstinate psoriatic lesions ($D_{1/2}$, 1–3 mm; HVL, up to 0.2 mm Al; TSD 15–30 cm; dosage, 3 $\times$ 100 R).

Scalp.   Because of the risk of a cumulative effect on the hair papilla, which may result in temporary alopecia, other therapeutic methods are preferred.

Face.   Small isolated lesions of the face should be treated only in exceptional cases. In young patients, irradiation is contraindicated (see indications, p. 113).

Radiation quality.   Grenz rays are preferred.

Dosage.   With grenz rays, single doses of 100–250 R may be given about three times at weekly intervals, up to a total of 300–750 R. The course may be repeated once after 4 weeks. Not more than two or three series per lesion should be given in a lifetime (Witten 1960). With grenz ray qualities, the maximum cumulative dose per area should not exceed 5,000 R (Pillsbury et al. 1956).

Anogenital region.   Radiotherapy is indicated only in very rare cases, and then only in older patients.

Radiation quality.   Grenz rays are favored.

Dosage.   Single doses of 100–250 R may be administered three or four times at weekly intervals.

Palms and soles.   Lesions in this location represent a limited indication for radiotherapy (for contraindications, see p. 125).

Radiation quality.   Soft x rays having a $D_{1/2}$ of 3–4 mm (HVL, 0.2 mm Al; TSD, 15–30 cm) are preferred.

Dosage.   Single doses of 75–80 R may be given two to four times at weekly intervals. Grenz rays are effective only when higher individual doses are used (250–300 R).

Therapeutic results.   The lesions involute rapidly. Recurrences may be expected.

Nails. X rays have been employed in the treatment of psoriatic nail changes because other forms of therapy are largely ineffective.

Radiation quality. X rays with a $D_{1/2}$ of 3–8 mm (HVL, 0.2–0.4 mm Al; TSD, 15–30 cm) are preferred.

Dosage. Single doses of 100–150 R are delivered three times at weekly intervals to the nails and paronychial tissue (matrix and nail bed). The maximum permissible dose (1,000 R per area and lifetime) must not be exceeded.

Therapeutic results. The morbidistatic effect of x rays is not apparent until several weeks after treatment. Favorable results have been reported in about two-thirds of the patients treated but recurrences may be expected. The failure to control recurrence clearly illustrates the dilemma one faces in using x rays in the treatment of benign recurrent dermatoses.

PUSTULAR PSORIASIS
The response of the various types of pustular psoriasis to x rays is so unpredictable that this form of therapy is not advised.

GENERALIZED PSORIASIS VULGARIS, PSORIATIC ERYTHRODERMA

Most authors agree that radiation treatment of psoriasis vulgaris in patients younger than 50–60 years should be limited to psoriatic erythroderma. Patients with recalcitrant erythroderma and generalized psoriasis vulgaris refractory to other forms of therapy are candidates for this treatment.

Radiation quality. Teleroentgen therapy has proved to be the most suitable method for this condition. Whole body irradiation is given at 50 kV without filter ($D_{1/2}$, 2 mm; TSD, 2 m; HVL, 0.1 mm Al). Shielding of the gonads is imperative. During radiation therapy, treatment with potentially irritating topical agents (tar, anthralin, etc.) should be suspended.

Dosage. Depending on the stage of the disease, single doses of 50 R are delivered every other day to the frontal or dorsal body surface, or to both. The total dosage is 350–500 R for generalized psoriasis, 400–550 R for psoriatic erythroderma.

Therapeutic results. In the majority of the patients treated, good results have been obtained even in severe cases of long standing. Frequently, the disease becomes again manageable by topical remedies after teleroentgen therapy.

PARAPSORIASIS GROUP

Radiation treatment is not indicated in pityriasis lichenoides chronica (parapsoriasis guttata), pityriasis lichenoides et varioliformis acuta (Mucha–Habermann), parakeratosis variegata (parapsoriasis lichenoides), and Brocq's disease (parapsoriasis en plaques). A favorable response to radiation therapy can be expected only in pre-mycosis fungoides lesions.

LICHEN PLANUS

Radiotherapy of lichen planus is limited to exceptional highly pruritic cases.

Indication. In most instances this benign dermatosis can be treated by other therapeutic means. Radiotherapy is justified only in intractable, highly pruritic localized lesions. Postradiation recurrences are less frequent than in psoriasis. In acute widespread lichen planus, exacerbations have occurred occasionally following radiation treatment (Koebner effect). Hence, ionizing radiation should be avoided in this type of lichen planus.

The decision to use x rays in the treatment of lichen planus should be based on the following criteria:

1. Use radiotherapy only in cases not amenable to other forms of therapy.
2. Confine radiotherapy to severely itching lesions, utilizing the marked antipruritic effect of x rays.
3. Do not use x rays in areas of cosmetic importance; they have a tendency to enhance the hyperpigmentation often seen in healing lesions of lichen planus.
4. Do not irradiate acute exanthematous eruptions (Koebner effect).
5. Do not use radiotherapy in children or adolescents.

Radiation quality. Depending on the depth of the lesions, grenz rays or soft x rays may be indicated ($D_{1/2}$, 2–4 mm; HVL, 0.2 mm Al; TSD, 15–30 cm).

Dosage. When grenz rays are used, single doses of 100–250 R may be given at weekly intervals, to a total of 1,200–2,000 R.

With soft x rays, individual doses of 60–100 R are administered. Total dose per course of treatment is 300–400 R; two or three courses may be given in a lifetime (maximum permissible dose per area, 1,000 R).

Therapeutic results. Rapid improvement has been observed but recurrences may occur. Hyperpigmentation often follows radiotherapy.

LICHEN PLANUS VERRUCOSUS (Hypertrophic Lichen Planus)

Radiation treatment should be tried only in persistent, refractory cases associated with severe pruritus.

Radiation quality. Depending on the depth of the lesions, soft x rays having a $D_{1/2}$ of 3–6 mm (HVL, 0.2–0.4 mm Al; TSD, 15–30 cm) are indicated.

Dosage. Single doses of 100–200 R may be administered weekly, up to a total of 300–600 R. The maximum permissible dose (1,000 R per area and lifetime) must not be exceeded.

Therapeutic results. Moderate to good results have been reported.

LICHEN PLANUS OF THE MUCOUS MEMBRANES

There is no indication for radiotherapy with this condition.

Dyskeratoses

KERATOSIS FOLLICULARIS (Darier's Disease)

In cases where all available therapeutic measures have been unsuccessful, a trial with x rays may be justified. The criteria listed under "Indications for Radiotherapy of Dermatoses" (p. 113) must be observed carefully.

Radiation quality. Grenz rays ($D_{1/2}$, 0.5 mm; HVL, 0.03 mm Al) are adequate for most cases (Hollander 1968).

Dosage. Although some authors have advocated low single doses of grenz rays (100 R four to six times at weekly intervals), a higher dosage (four to six single doses of 200–400 R at 2–3 week intervals) is more likely to influence this disorder.

Therapeutic results. Alleviation of pruritus, remissions, and even permanent cures have been reported. Only circumscribed lesions appear to be suitable for this treatment.

Granulomatous Diseases of the Skin

SARCOIDOSIS (Boeck's Sarcoid)

Radiotherapy is rarely successful in this disease. (Some authors recommend soft x-ray qualities: HVL, 0.4 mm Al; TSD, 30 cm; $D_{1/2}$, 7 mm; dosage: single fractions of 300 R daily, to a total of 3,000 R or more). Radiation sequelae should be expected with higher doses.

GRANULOMA ANNULARE

There is no clear indication for radiotherapy; small doses of grenz rays are occasionally helpful.

EOSINOPHILIC GRANULOMA OF THE SKIN

This disorder is largely radioresistant. Recently, however, there have been reports on successful treatment with soft x rays, especially in the tumorous type of eosinophilic granuloma.

Radiation quality. Radiation having a $D_{1/2}$ of 3–10 mm (HVL, 0.2–0.5 mm Al; TSD, 30 cm) has been recommended. Occasionally, x rays with a $D_{1/2}$ of 3 cm (intermediate therapy) have been used.

Dosage. In the tumorous variety, single fractions of 200 R are given, up to a total of 1,000–2,400 R (more in isolated cases).

GRANULOMA FACIALE (Eosinophilic Granuloma of the Face)

Ionizing radiation is used occasionally with good results.

Radiation quality. Soft x rays with a $D_{1/2}$ of 3–10 mm (HVL, 0.2–0.5 mm Al; TSD, 30 cm) are recommended.

Dosage. Single fractions of 200 R are administered in the course of 4 months, to a total of 2,000 R.

Therapeutic results. The lesions are relatively radioresistant. Other therapeutic measures should be tried before radiotherapy is used.

Diseases of the Connective Tissue

POIKILODERMA VASCULARE ATROPHICANS

There is no indication for radiotherapy with this condition.

LICHEN SCLEROSUS ET ATROPHICUS (Kraurosis Vulvae)

Application of radiotherapy in this disorder is controversial (see p. 103).

LUPUS ERYTHEMATOSUS

CHRONIC DISCOID LUPUS ERYTHEMATOSUS

Radiotherapy is contraindicated because of the risk of exacerbation.

DUPUYTREN'S CONTRACTURE

This hereditary fibromatosis of the palmar aponeurosis occurs almost exclusively in males and is sometimes associated with plastic induration of the penis. It eventually produces disabling contractures.

Radiotherapy is indicated only in the early stage of the disease. Cases where marked contractures are already present should not be treated.

Technique. The surrounding tissue must be thoroughly shielded. The central beam should not be directed toward the gonads. The patient should be treated in a sitting position, with his hand positioned on an x-ray table covered with lead rubber.

Radiation quality. Superficial x-ray therapy is the method of choice. The radiation quality ($D_{1/2}$, 12–15 mm; HVL, 0.8–1.4 mm Al; TSD, 15 cm; filter, 2 mm Al and 2 mm Cellon) is the same as that employed in plastic induration of the penis (see below). More penetrating radiation is not advised. An additional filter of 2-mm thickness of a tissue-equivalent material (Cellon) is recommended to eliminate softer x rays, which may unnecessarily damage unaffected superficial skin layers.

Dosage. Single doses of 400 R are administered on two consecutive days. A maximum total dosage of 2,400 R may be given, with 8–10 week intervals between treatments. If the disease responds to the treatment, improvement is seen after 2,400 R; higher doses are not advised because of the increased risk of late sequelae.

Therapeutic results. If treated in its early stages, the disease may be arrested or even cured. In the late stages, only surgical treatment is indicated.

PLASTIC INDURATION OF THE PENIS (Peyronie's Disease)

This fibromatosis originates in the tunica albuginea and causes pain and curvature of the penis on erection. Not infrequently, this disorder is associated with Dupuytren's contracture, fibrosis mammae virilis, and keloids (polyfibromatosis of Touraine). Radiotherapy is of little or no benefit, particularly in cases where calcareous deposits in the lesions can be demonstrated radiologically.

Disturbances of Pigmentation

VITILIGO

Radiotherapy is not indicated in this disorder. Therapeutic results are difficult to evaluate because of spontaneous improvement.

131

Diseases of the Sebaceous Glands

ACNE VULGARIS

Radiotherapy of acne vulgaris now is reserved for rare, extremely severe cases. Its beneficial effect results from a temporary reduction in size of the sebaceous glands and reduced sebum production (Strauss and Kligman 1959). Satisfactory long-term results have been reported (Epstein, 1971 a) but recurrences cannot always be avoided. The following criteria should be observed:

1. Use only in extremely severe cases refractory to other types of therapy.
2. Use only in patients over 17 years of age.
3. Do not use in fair-skinned, blue-eyed, and red-haired patients.
4. Do not use in drug-induced or occupational forms of acne.
5. Insure protection of radiosensitive organs (gonads, eyes, thyroid).
6. Never exceed the maximum permissible dose of 1,000 R per area and lifetime.

Radiation quality. Superficial x rays with a $D_{1/2}$ of 4–8 mm (HVL, 0.7 mm Al; TSD, 30 cm) have been advocated. Cones should be used for radiation protection and the beam should be centered to the zygomatic areas.

Dosage. Single doses of 60–85 R are given to either cheek (and forehead) at weekly intervals, to a total of 600–800 R.

Therapeutic results. The therapeutic efficacy of radiation therapy is uncontested and can be proved histologically. After 6 months, the sebaceous glands gradually return to their original size and recurrences may occur. However, other forms of treatment are often more effective following a course of radiotherapy.

Diseases of the Apocrine Sweat Glands

FOX–FORDYCE DISEASE

Indication. Radiotherapy may be indicated in exceptional, severely pruritic, refractory cases.

Radiation quality. X rays with a $D_{1/2}$ of 4–10 mm (HVL, 0.2–0.5 mm Al; TSD, 15–30 cm) may be used.

Dosage.   Single doses of 100–400 R may be given at 1–8 day intervals, up to a total of 800 R (maximum dose per field: 1,000 R).

Diseases of the Eccrine Sweat Glands

LOCALIZED HYPERHIDROSIS

The radiation doses required to produce a therapeutic effect are high enough to cause late sequelae. This treatment is therefore no longer advocated.

Disorders of the Hair

HYPERTRICHOSIS

Permanent x-ray epilation is no longer used because the necessary high radiation doses may induce severe radiation damage. Many cases of chronic radiodermatitis have resulted from indiscriminate epilation treatments by laymen (Tricho Institutes) for facial hypertrichosis in women.

Diseases of the Nails

Limited indications for radiotherapy include paronychia (p. 119), onychodystrophy secondary to eczema (p. 123), and psoriatic nail changes (p. 127).

Teleroentgen therapy
of generalized dermatoses

6.1   GENERAL CONSIDERATIONS

Teleroentgen therapy (Schirren 1955, 1959 b) is used for the treatment of the entire body surface, particularly in chronic generalized dermatoses. The advantages of the method may be summarized as follows (Gold-schmidt 1962; Lukacs and Goldschmidt, in press):

1. The radiation dose exerts its full effect on the pathologic process; the skin is irradiated uniformly.
2. The rapid falloff of the radiation protects normal under-lying tissue.
3. There are no systemic effects.

Teleroentgen therapy was impractical as long as only glass-windowed tubes with a low dose rate were available. Introduction of the beryllium-window tube has made it possible to utilize the range of radiation qualities between grenz rays and 50 kV, which is particularly suited to dermatologic radiation therapy.

6.2   PHYSICAL FOUNDATION
OF TELEROENTGEN THERAPY

Irradiation of the entire body surface (frontal or dorsal aspect) as a single field requires a TSD of 2 m. At this distance, the dose rate of unfiltered radiation produced at 50 kV is about 20 R/min. The usually very high dose rate close to the window is reduced markedly at a distance of 2 m because the air acts as a filter for very soft x rays, which comprise a major portion of the x-ray beam.

Distribution of the Dose Rate

When the central beam is aimed at a point between umbilicus and symphysis pubis, the skin of the trunk, arms, and thighs of a patient of average height positioned at a distance of 2 m receives relatively uniform irradiation (see Fig. 38 on p. 97). The radiation intensity at the periphery (head and lower legs) measures approximately 70% of the central beam.

Depth of Penetration

The dosage falloff of unfiltered radiation from a beryllium tube is largely independent of voltage but is greatly dependent on long target–skin distance because of the degree of absorption in air. At a distance of 2 m, without filtration, the $D_{1/2}$ at 50 kV (25 mA) is 2 mm.

6.3 RADIATION PROTECTION IN TELEROENTGEN THERAPY

Despite the rapid falloff of the radiation dose in the skin, small doses may reach the underlying tissue; e.g., if the frontal body surface is irradiated with a total dose of 1,000 R and only a simple lead shield is used to protect the gonads, 45 R will penetrate to underlying tissue. Protection of the gonads is therefore of utmost importance. Male patients should wear a tightly fitting, 1-mm thick lead bag that completely encloses the genitals and is fastened around the waist (see Fig. 38). This should be worn when the anterior as well as the posterior surface is treated. In female patients, satisfactory protection is achieved by using 20 × 15 cm lead shields both on the anterior and posterior aspects of the body at the level of the ovaries. Although the gonadal dose is very small (only 75 mR per 1,000 R in male patients wearing a lead bag) teleroentgen therapy should be used judiciously, especially in patients of reproductive age. In this group, the method is indicated only as a last resort in life-threatening diseases (e.g., mycosis fungoides) after other therapeutic alternatives have been exhausted. Compared to the gonad dose delivered to the ovaries during intravenous pyelog-

136

raphy (290 mR), the gonad dose for teleroentgen therapy with a total dose of 500 R to anterior and posterior surfaces is only 425 mR if proper protection is used. Shielding of the eyes is also very important.

Radiation Protection for Medical Personnel

Because the amount of backscatter encountered with this method considerably exceeds normal limits, a treatment room equipped with structural shielding (leaded walls) and a built–in therapy unit operated from a panel outside the room is desirable. Adequate ventilation is also essential. Because of these requirements, teleroentgen therapy is usually performed only in hospitals.

6.4 TECHNICAL PROCEDURE

The procedure is illustrated schematically in Fig. 38 for unfiltered beryllium tube radiation with a TSD of 2 m (50 kV; 25 mA; no filter; $D_{1/2}$, 2 mm). Lead shielding of gonads and eyes is imperative. Grab bars and backrest can be used as steadying devices.

Dosage

Single doses vary with the stage of the pathologic process—the more acute the disorder, the smaller the dose. In benign generalized dermatoses or erythroderma, single doses may vary from 30 to 50 R, given at 2-day intervals to either or both body surfaces, up to a total of 300–600 R. In malignant diseases (e.g., mycosis fungoides, malignant lymphomas), single doses of 50–80 R may be administered daily, to a total of 1,000–1,500 R. While hematopoietic changes have not been reported with this method, periodic blood counts are advisable. Systemic effects have not been observed.

6.5 INDICATIONS FOR
TELEROENTGEN THERAPY

PRURITUS

Indication. Intractable nonspecific senile pruritus is amenable to teleroentgen therapy when other therapeutic methods have failed.

Dosage. Single doses of 50 R may be administered at 2-day intervals to either or both body surfaces, up to a total of 300–600 R.

Therapeutic results. Good results have been obtained.

ERYTHRODERMA SECONDARY TO LICHEN PLANUS

Stubborn, widespread lesions of lichen planus may be suitable for teleroentgen therapy; contraindications should be observed carefully.

Dosage. Every other day, 50 R may be given to each aspect of the body surface; the total dose generally ranges from 400 to 500 R.

Therapeutic results. Improvement usually becomes manifest after a few treatments; itching is controlled promptly. Subsequent hyperpigmentation is not uncommon.

PSORIASIS VULGARIS

Indication. In generalized psoriasis or psoriatic erythroderma not responsive to other forms of therapy, a trial with teleroentgen therapy may be indicated.

Dosage. The frontal and dorsal aspects of the body surface may be treated alternately or simultaneously with single doses of 30–50 R at 2–3 day intervals, to a total of 350–500 R. Bland concomitant topical treatments (vaseline, corticosteroid ointments) are advised; coal tar or anthraline should be avoided.

Therapeutic results. Favorable results have been obtained even with small doses.

ERYTHRODERMA SECONDARY TO OTHER DERMATOSES

Erythroderma associated with dermatoses other than psoriasis (e.g., pityriasis rubra pilaris) may also benefit from teleroentgen therapy.

Dosage. Single doses of 30–50 R are given on alternate days to either one or both aspects of the body, up to a total of 500–600 R.

Therapeutic results. Significant improvement is obtained in the majority of the cases. Refractory erythroderma frequently becomes manageable by local measures after teleroentgen therapy. Relapses are, of course, unavoidable.

GENERALIZED ECZEMATOUS DERMATITIS

Indication. Teleroentgen therapy is justified in cases of generalized eczema not responsive to other forms of therapy. Different types of eczema respond equally well to this method.

Dosage. Single doses of 50 R are given at 2-day intervals, to a total of 400–600 R.

Therapeutic results. The results are good, but careful selection of the cases is essential.

MYCOSIS FUNGOIDES

Indication. The plaque stage and the erythrodermic variety are well suited for teleroentgen therapy. In the tumor stage better results are obtained with electron beam treatments.

Dosage. Fifty to 100 R are given daily or at 2-day intervals to the anterior and posterior surface of the body. The total dose will vary from 500 to 1,000 R. In view of the potential serious nature of the disease, treatment courses of 500–800 R can be repeated several times at 2–3 month intervals. Telangiectases and other evidence of chronic radiodermatitis are possible after 2,000–3,000 R.

Therapeutic results. Erythema and residual pigmentation will subside after several weeks. Pruritus is alleviated promptly. Lesions irradiated previously often involute more slowly. As with other treatment modalities, the effect of treatment is palliative, not curative. Regular blood counts are imperative, especially if cytotoxic drugs are given concurrently.

ERYTHRODERMA OF THE AGED, ASSOCIATED WITH CACHEXIA AND LYMPHADENOPATHY

This syndrome is well suited for palliative teleroentgen therapy.

Dosage. Single doses of 50 R are given on alternate days to one or both aspects of the body, up to a total of 300–500 R.

Therapeutic results. Teleroentgen therapy produces favorable results in combination with systemic corticosteroid and/or cytotoxic treatment. Despite alleviation of the cutaneous manifestations, the prognosis remains unchanged.

bibliography

Arma-Szlachcic, M., F. Ott, and H. Storck. Zur Strahlentherapie der mela-
notischen Präcancerosen. *Hautarzt* 21: 505–508, 1970.

Baer, R.L., and Kopf, A.W. Complications of therapy of basal cell epitheliomas, *Year Book of Dermatology*, 7–26. Chicago: Year Book
Medical Publishers, 1965.

Baer, R.L., and Witten, V.H. Selected aspects of dermatologic therapy
with superficial x rays and grenz rays, *Year Book of Dermatology*,
7–35. Chicago: Year Book Medical Publishers, 1956.

Barth, G. Nahbestrahlung. In: Handbuch der medizinischen Radiologie,
Vol. XVI/1, Hug, O. (ed.). Berlin, Heidelberg, New York, Springer-
Verlag, 1970.

Barth, R.S., Kopf, A.W., and Petratos, M.A. X-ray therapy of skin cancer:
Evaluation of a "standardized" method for treating basal cell epithe-
liomas. *Proc. Sixth National Cancer Conference, 1968.* Philadelphia:
J.B. Lippincott, 1969.

Bode, H.G. Strahlentherapie von Hautkrankheiten. In: *Haut- und Geschlechtskrankheiten*, Vol. II, A. 764–790, H.G. Bode and G.W.
Korting (eds.). Stuttgart: Fischer, 1970.

Braun-Falco, O., Lukacs, S., and Schoefinius, H.H. Zur Behandlung der
Melanosis circumscripta praecancerosa Dubreuilh. *Hautarzt* 26:
207–210, 1975.

Chaoul, H. *Die Nahbestrahlung.* Stuttgart: Georg Thieme, 1943.

Chaoul, H., and Wachsmann, F. *Die Nahbestrahlung,* 2nd ed. Stuttgart: Thieme, 1953.

Cipollaro, A.C., and Crossland, P.M. X rays and Radium in the Treatment of Diseases of the Skin, 5th ed. Philadelphia: Lea & Febiger, 1967.

Domonkos, A.N. *Andrews' Diseases of the Skin,* Phildelphia: W.B. Saunders, 1971.

Domonkos, A.N. Treatment of eyelid carcinoma, *Arch. Dermatol.* 91: 364–370, 1965.

Du Mesnil de Rochemont, R. *Lehrbuch der Strahlenheilkunde.* Stuttgart: Enke, 1958.

Epstein, E. Radiodermatitis. Springfield, Ill.: Charles C Thomas, 1962.

Epstein, E. Dermatologic radiotherapy, 1965. *Arch. Dermatol.* 92: 307–314, 1965.

Epstein, E. X-ray therapy in acne, *Cutis* 8: 321, 1971.

Epstein, E. Radiation therapy of benign dermatoses. *Dermatol. Digest,* 39, 1971b.

Epstein, E.V., Levin, D.L., Croft, J.D., and Lutzner, M.A. Mycosis fungoides. *Medicine* 15: 61, 1972.

Franke, H.D. Die Anwendung strahlensensibilisierender Substanzen in der Strahlentherapie. *Strahlentherapie* 143: 296, 1972.

Freeman, R.G., and Knox, J.M.: *Treatment of Skin Cancer.* New York: Springer-Verlag, 1967.

Fritz-Niggli, H. *Strahlenbiologie und Ergebnisse.* Stuttgart: Thieme, 1959.

Fromer, J.L., Johnston, D.O., and Salzman, F.A. Management of lymphoma cutis with low megavolt electron beam therapy: Nine year follow-up in 200 cases. *South. Med J.* 54: 769, 1961.

Fuks, Z., and Bagshaw, M.A. Total-skin electron treatment of mycosis fungoides, *Radiology* 100: 145, 1971.

Gahlen, W. Weichstrahltherapie. In: *Handbuch der medizinischen Radiologie,* Vol. XVI/1. Berlin, Heidelberg, New York: Springer-Verlag, 1970.

Gladstein, A.H. Modification of eye shields for use in x-ray therapy of eyelid cancers. *Arch. Dermatol.* 110: 793, 1974.

Gladstein, A.H. Radiation protection. In: *Physical Modalities in Dermatologic Therapy.* Goldschmidt, H. (ed.). New York-Berlin-Heidelberg: Springer-Verlag (in press).

Goldschmidt, H. Die Roentgentherapie von Dermatosen. In: *Handbuch der Haut- und Geschlechtskrankheiten.* Suppl. Vol. V/2, Jadassohn, J. (ed.). Berlin: Springer, 1959, pp. 486–598.

Goldschmidt, H. Teleroentgen Irradiation in Dermatologic Therapy. Low Voltage (Soft X rays). *Proc. XII Int. Cong. Dermatol. Washing-*

ton, D.C., 1962, Vol. 1. Amsterdam: Excerpta Medica Foundation, 1962, p. 643.

Goldschmidt, H. X-ray Treatment of Skin Cancers. Proc. XIII Int. Cong. Dermatol., Munich, 1967. Berlin: Springer, 1968, p. 105.

Goldschmidt, H. Gesichtspunkte zur Auswahl der Bestrahlungsbedingungen. In: *Fortschritte der praktischen Dermatologie und Venerologie*, Braun-Falco, O. and Petzold, D. (eds.). Berlin: Springer-Verlag, 1973, p. 298–305.

Goldschmidt, H. Radiotherapy of skin cancer. *Cutis* 17: 253–261, 1976.

Goldschmidt, H. Dermatologic radiation therapy. Current use of ionizing radiation in the United States and Canada. *Arch. Dermatol.* 111: 1511–1517, 1975.

Goldschmidt, H. Dermatologic radiation therapy. In: *Dermatology*, Moschella, S., Pillsbury, D.M., and Hurley, H.J. (eds.). Philadelphia: Saunders: 1975, p. 1664–1690.

Goldschmidt, H. Dermatologic radiotherapy: Selection of radiation qualities and treatment techniques. *Int. J. Dermatol.* 15: 171–181, 1976.

Goldschmidt, H. (ed.) *Physical Modalities in Dermatologic Therapy*. New York-Berlin-Heidelberg: Springer-Verlag (in press).

Gorson, R.O. Physical aspects of dermatologic radiotherapy. In: *Physical Modalities in Dermatologic Therapy*. Goldschmidt, H. (ed.). New York-Berlin-Heidelberg: Springer-Verlag (in press).

Grover, R.W. In: *Radiotherapy of benign diseases*, S.B. Dewing (ed.). Springfield, Ill.: Charles C Thomas, 1965.

Harber, L.E. Clinical evaluation of radiation therapy in psoriasis. *Arch. Dermatol.* 77: 554, 1958.

Hauss, H., Proppe, A., and Goldschmidt, H. Radiotherapy of lentigo maligna and Bowen's disease. In: *Physical Modalities in Dermatologic Therapy*, Goldschmidt, H. (ed.). New York-Berlin-Heidelberg: Springer-Verlag (in press).

Hollander, M.B. *Ultra Soft X rays*. Baltimore: Williams & Wilkins Co., 1968.

Hornstein, O.P. Therapie und Prognose des malignen Melanoms. *Fortschr. Med.* 90: 1087, 1972.

Hug, O., and Trott, K.R. In: *Kernenergie, Nutzen und Risiko*, K. H. Lindackers (ed.). Stuttgart: DVA, 1970.

Jennings, W.A.: Low voltage x-ray therapy with a beryllium window tube. Part II. The achievement of optimum depth dosage distributions— from the physical standpoint. *Br. J. Radiol.* 24: 135, 1951.

Johns, H.E., and Cunningham, J.R. *The Physics of Radiology*, 3rd ed., Springfield, Ill.: Charles C Thomas, 1969.

Keining, E., and Braun-Falco, O. *Dermatologie und Venerologie*. München: J.F. Lehmann, 1970.

Knierer, W., and Schirren, C.G. Eine neue Art von Augenschutzschalen. *Strahlentherapie* 89: 606, 1953.

Knight, A.G. Grenz ray therapy of herpes simplex. *Br. J. Dermatol.* 86: 172, 1972.

Kopf, A.W. Therapy of basal cell carcinoma. In: *Dermatology in General Medicine*, Arndt, K.A., Clark, W.H., Eisen, A.Z., Van Scott, E.J., and Vaughan, J.H. (eds). New York: McGraw-Hill Book Co., 1971, p. 472–490.

Kopf, A.W., Bart, R.S., and Gladstein, A.H. Treatment of melanotic freckle with x rays. *Arch Dermatol.* 112: 801–807, 1976.

Lorenz, W. *Strahlenschutz in Klinik und ärztlicher Praxis.* Stuttgart: Thieme, 1961.

Lukacs, S. Häufige röntgentherapeutische Indikationen. In: *Fortschritte der praktischen Dermatologie und Venerologie*, Braun-Falco, O., and Petzold, D. (eds.). Berlin: Springer-Verlag, 1973.

Lukacs, S., and Goldschmidt, H. Teleroentgentherapy of mycosis fungoides and benign dermatoses. In: *Physical Modalities in Dermatologic Therapy*, Goldschmidt, H. (ed.). New York-Berlin-Heidelberg: Springer-Verlag (in press).

Miescher, G. Über Klinik und Therapie der Melanome. *Arch. Dermatol. Syph.* (Berl.) 200: 215, 1955.

Modan, B., Baldatz, D., Mart, H., Steinitz, R., and Levin, S.R. Radiation-induced head and neck tumors. *Lancet* 1: 277, 1974.

Petratos, M.A., Kopf, A.W., Bart, R.B., Grisewood, E.N., and Gladstein, A.H.: Treatment of Melanotic Freckles with X rays. *Arch. Dermatol.*, 106: 189–194, 1972.

Pillsbury, D.M. Use and abuse of x-ray therapy for benign skin conditions. *Postgrad. Med. J.*, 30: 180, 1961.

Pillsbury, D.M., Shelley, W.B., and Kligman, A.M. *Dermatology.* Philadelphia: Saunders, 1956.

Pipkin, J.L., Lehmann, C.F., and Ressman, A. Treatment of plantar warts by single dose method of roentgen ray. *South. Med. J.* 42: 193, 1949.

Proppe, A. Spezielle Röntgen-Behandlung. In: *Dermatologie und Venerologie*, Vol. II/1, Gottron, H.A. and Schönfeld W. (ed.). Stuttgart: Thieme, 1958.

Rajewsky, B., and Pohlit, W. Strahlenschäden und Strahlenschutz. In: *Handbuch der Haut- und Geschlechtskrankheiten*, Suppl. Vol. V/2, Jadassohn, J. (ed.). Berlin, Göttingen, Heidelberg: Springer-Verlag, 1959.

Rudolph, R., and Goldschmidt, H.: Radiodermatitis and other adverse sequelae of cutaneous irradiation. In: *Physical Modalities in Dermatologic Therapy.* Goldschmidt, H. (ed.). New York-Berlin-Heidelberg: Springer-Verlag (in press).

Scherer, E. *Strahlentherapie.* Stuttgart: Thieme, 1967.

Schirren, C.G. Roentgen irradiation at a distance using the soft radiation from beryllium window tubes in treating cases of generalized dermatoses. *J. Invest. Dermatol.,* 24: 463, 1955.

Schirren, C.G. Behandlung benigner und maligner Hautgeschwülste unter besonderer Berücksichtigung der Strahlentherapie. In: *Handbuch der Haut- und Geschlechtskrankheiten,* Suppl. Vol. V/2, Jadassohn, J. (ed.). Berlin, Göttingen, Heidelberg: Springer-Verlag, 1959a.

Schirren, C.G. Totalbestrahlung, Röntgen-Fernbestrahlung der Haut und indirekte Bestrahlungsmethoden. In: *Handbuch der Haut- und Geschlechtskrankheiten,* Suppl. Vol. V/2, Jadassohn, J. (ed.). Berlin, Göttingen, Heidelberg: Springer-Verlag, 1959b.

Schirren, C.G. Kritische Stellungnahme zur Anwendung radioaktiver Substanzen in der Therapie des praktischen Dermatologen, In: *Fortschritte der prakt. Dermatologie und Venerologie,* Vol. 4, Marchionini, A. (ed.). Berlin: Springer-Verlag, 1962, p. 259.

Schoefinius, H.H., Lukacs, S., and Braun-Falco, O. Zur Behandlung von Morbus Bowen, Bowen-Carcinom und Erythroplasie Queyrat unter besonderer Berücksichtigung der Roentgenweichstrahltherapie. *Hautarzt* 25: 489–493, 1974.

Selman, J. *The Basic Physics of Radiation Therapy.* Springfield, Ill.: Charles C Thomas, 1960.

Storck, H., Schwarz, K., and Ott, F. Haut. Intraepitheliale Carcinome. In: *Handbuch der medizinischen Radiologie,* Vol. XIX/1 S. 69, Diethelm, L., Olsson, O., Strnad, F., Vieten, H., and Zuppinger, A. (eds.). Berlin, Heidelberg, New York: Springer-Verlag, 1972.

Streffer, C. *Strahlen-Biochemie. Heidelberger Taschenbücher 59/60.* Berlin, Heidelberg, New York: Springer-Verlag, 1969.

Strauss, J.S., and Kligman, A.M. Effect of x rays on sebaceous glands of the human face; Radiation therapy of acne. *J. Invest. Dermatol.* 33: 347, 1959.

Sulzberger, M.B., Baer, R.L., and Borota, A. Do roentgen ray treatments as given by skin specialists produce cancers or other sequelae? *Arch. Dermatol.* 65: 639, 1952.

Trott, K.R. In: *Handbuch der medizinischen Radiologie,* Vol. II/3, Hug, O., and Zuppinger, A. (eds.). Berlin, Heidelberg, New York: Springer-Verlag, 1972.

Tuddenham, W.J. Half-value depth and fall-off-ratio as functions of portal area, target-skin distance and half-value layer. *Radiology* 69: 78, 1957.

van der Plaats, G.J. Die Kontaktbestrahlung. In: *Handbuch der medizinischen Radiologie,* Vol. XVI/1, Hug, O. (ed.). Berlin, Heidelberg, New York: Springer-Verlag, 1970.

van der Plaats, G.J. Die RöntgenKaustik, ihre Grundsätze und Anwendung. *Strahlentherapie* 61: 84, 1938.

Wachsmann, F. In: *Die Strahlentherapie; Physikalische Grundlagen der Röntgentherapie und Dosimetrie.* Meyer-Matthes, D. (ed.). Stuttgart: Georg Thieme, 1949.

Wachsmann, F. Allgemeine Methodik der Röntgentherapie von Hautkrankheiten. In: *Handbuch der Haut- und Geschlechtskrankheiten*, Suppl. Vol. V/2, Jadassohn, J. (ed.). Berlin, Göttingen, Heidelberg: Springer-Verlag, 1959.

Wachsmann, F., and Dimotsis, A. *Kurven und Tabellen für die Strahlentherapie.* Stuttgart: Hirzel, 1957.

Wachsmann, F., and Vieten, H. Grundlagen der strahlentherapeutischen Methoden. In: *Handbuch der medizinischen Radiologie; Allgemeine strahlentherapeutische Methodik*, Vol. XVI/1, Diethelm, L., Olsson, O., Strnad, F., Vieten, H., and Zuppinger, A. (eds.). Berlin, Heidelberg, New York: Springer-Verlag, 1970.

Wagner, G. Die Epilationsbestrahlung. In: *Handbuch der Haut- und Geschlechtskrankheiten, Ergänzungswerk*, Vol. V/2, Jadassohn, J. (ed.). Berlin-Göttingen-Heidelberg: Springer, 1959.

Walter, J., and Miller, H. *A Short Textbook of Radiotherapy.* London: J. and A. Churchill, Ltd., 1969.

Wiskemann, A. Strahlensensibilisierung mit Spindelgiften bei Mykosis fungoides. *Strahlentherapie* 143: 338, 1972.

Witten, V.H. Place of Grenz radiation in dermatologic practice. *Arch. Dermatol.* 81: 110, 1960.

Witten, V.H., and Kopf, A.W. Some common misconceptions regarding nevi and skin cancers. *Medical Clinics of North America* 43(3): 731–752, 1959.

Witten, V.H., Sulzberger, M.B., and Stewart, W.D. Studies on the quantity of radiation reaching the gonadal areas during dermatologic x-ray therapy. *Arch. Dermatol.* 76: 683–694, 1957.

Zoon, J.J., and Werz, J.F.C. The quality of x rays in the treatment of skin diseases. *Arch. Dermatol. Syph.* 75: 733, 1957.

index

146

Q

R

S

T